DEMENTIA
ACTIVITIES
FOR SENIORS

Dementia is a disease that makes an individual develop intellectual impairment as a result of changes in the brain. These include: problems with memory, orientation and counting. Dementia can be caused by natural aging process and genetic factors, other diseases and external factors. It is an incurable disease but you can counteract it or slow its progression. This book is intended for people who experience a decline in mental performance. The book is divided into 3 parts according to the degree of difficulty: easy, intermediate and difficult.

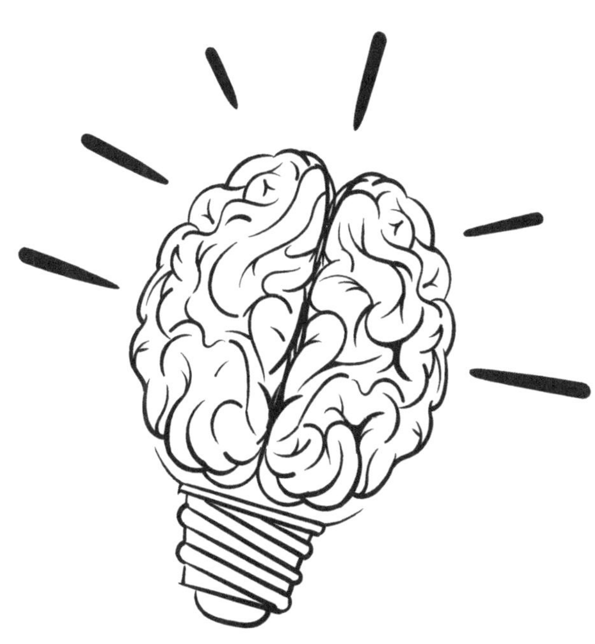

FELICIA AUSTIN

EASY LEVEL

1. Match pairs.

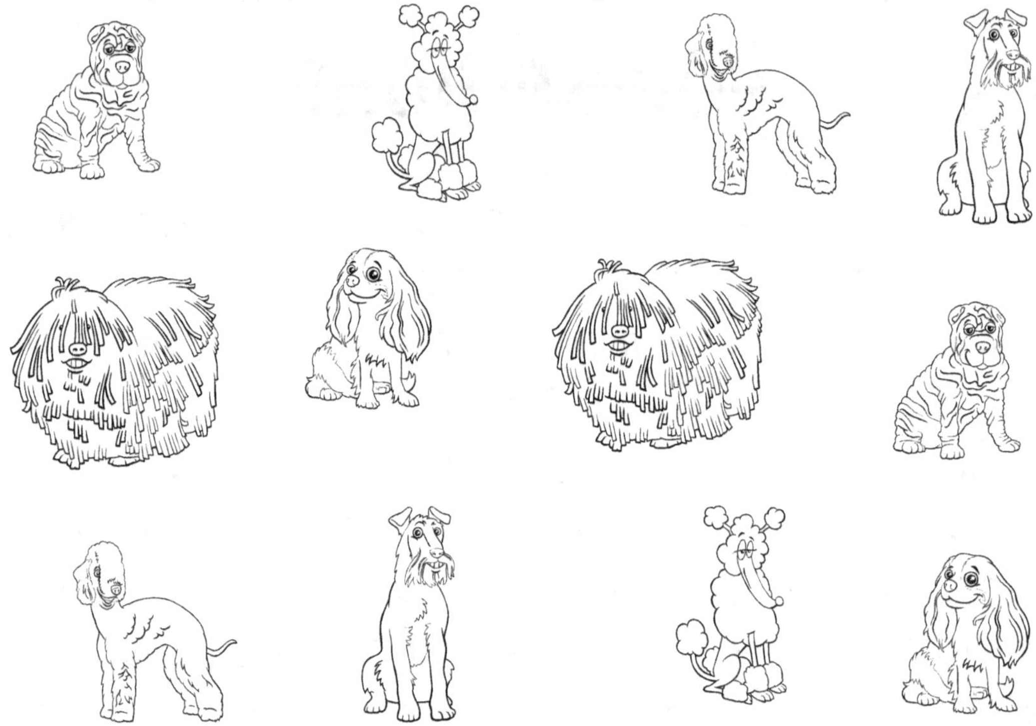

2. Copy the picture.

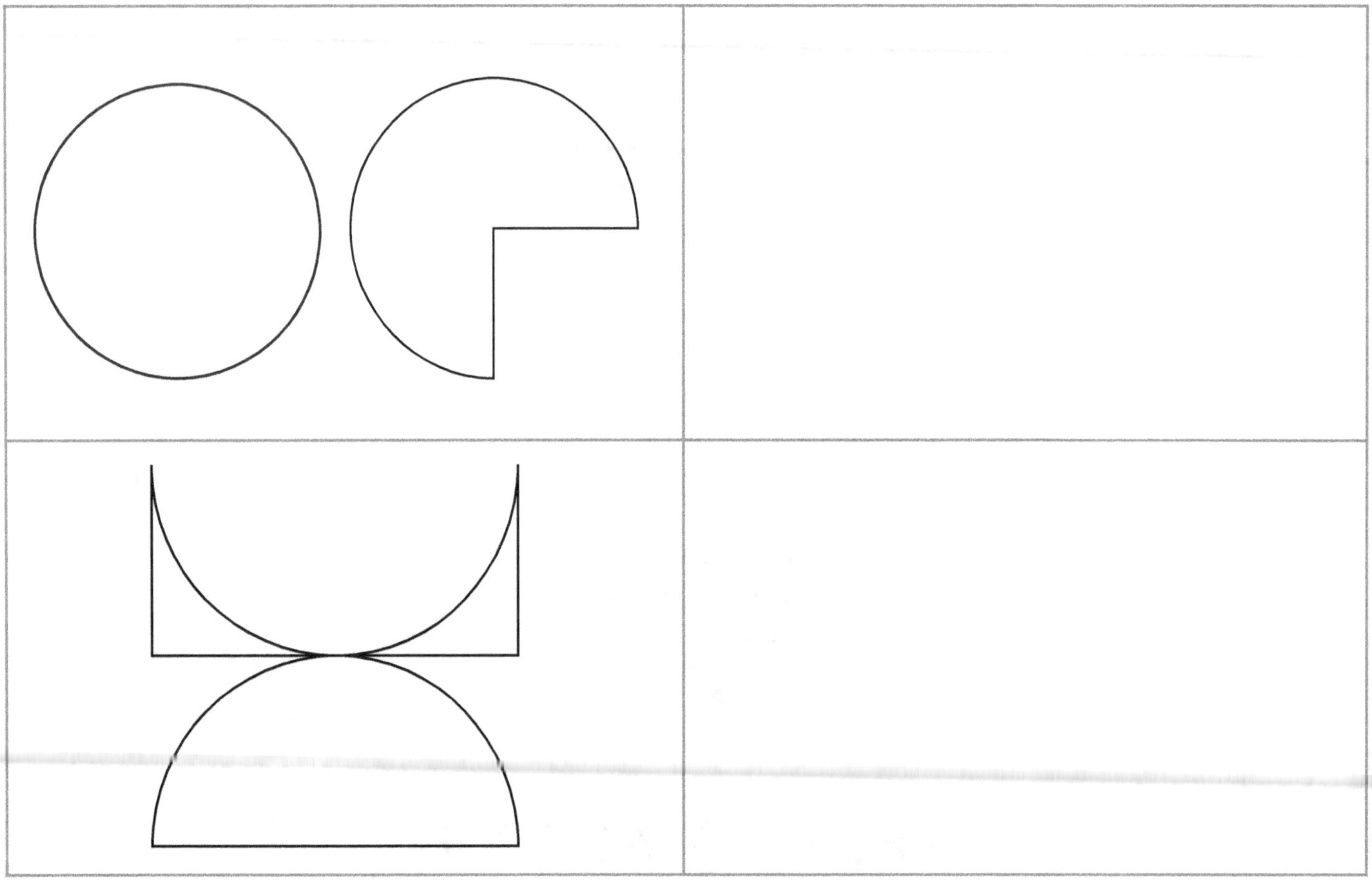

3. How many?

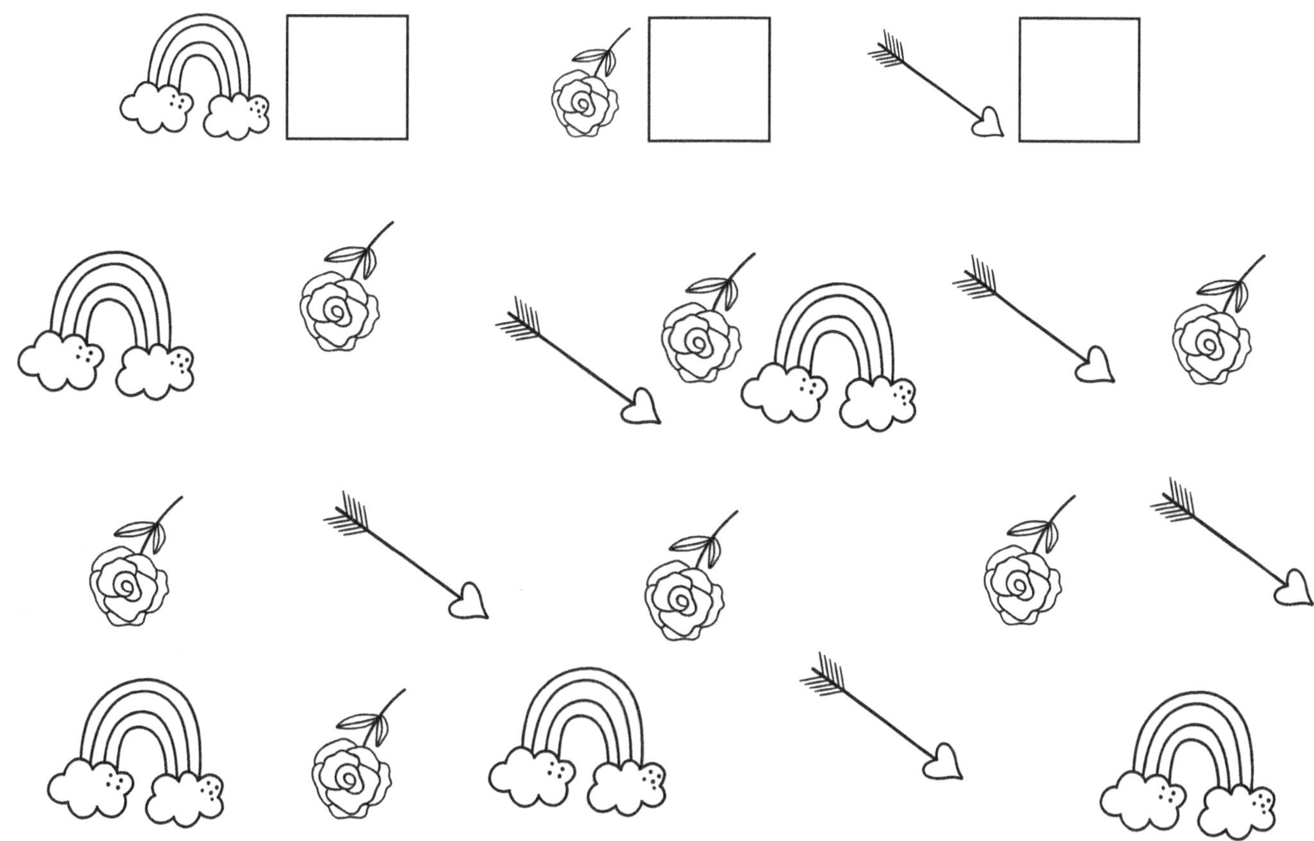

4. Find 5 differences

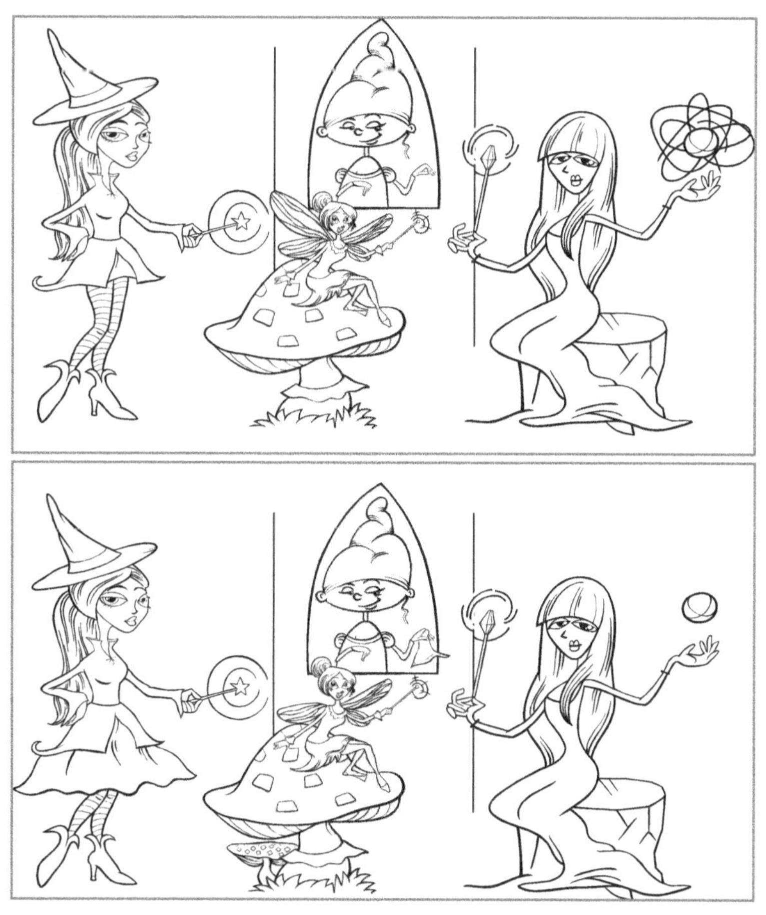

5. What would be useful on the beach?

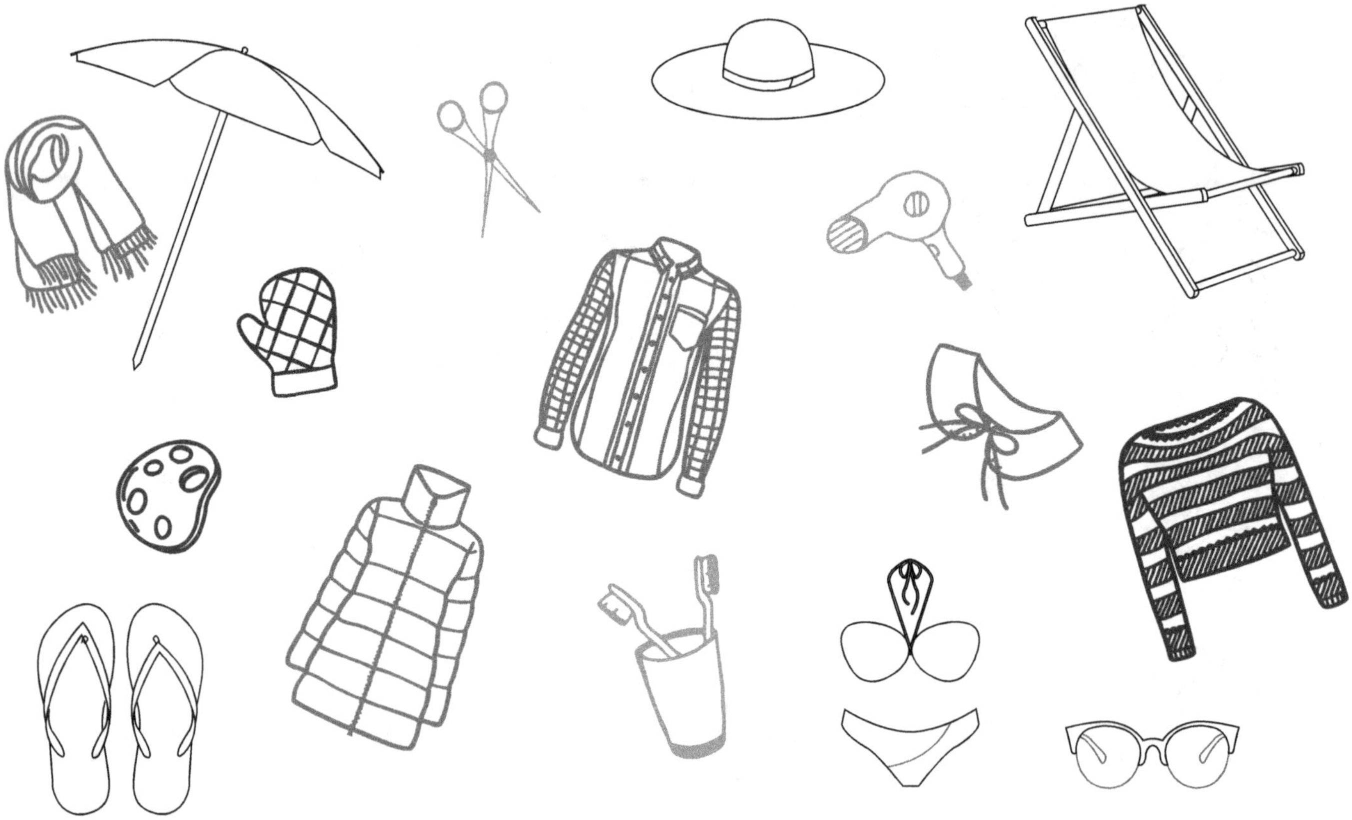

6. What does not fit?

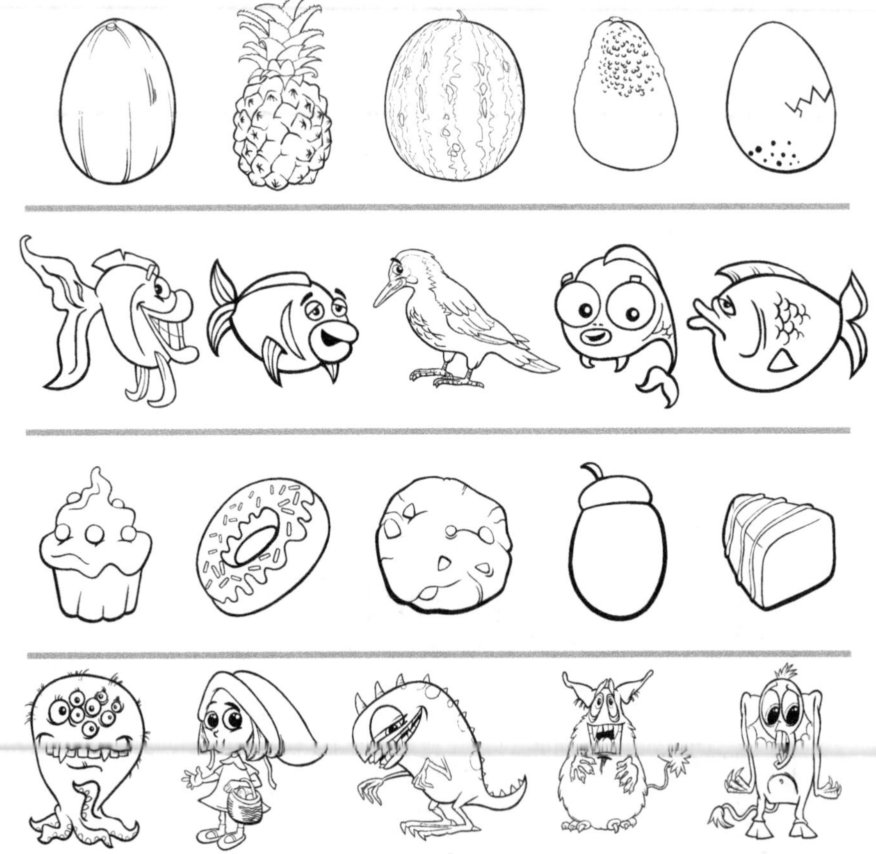

7. Matching game.

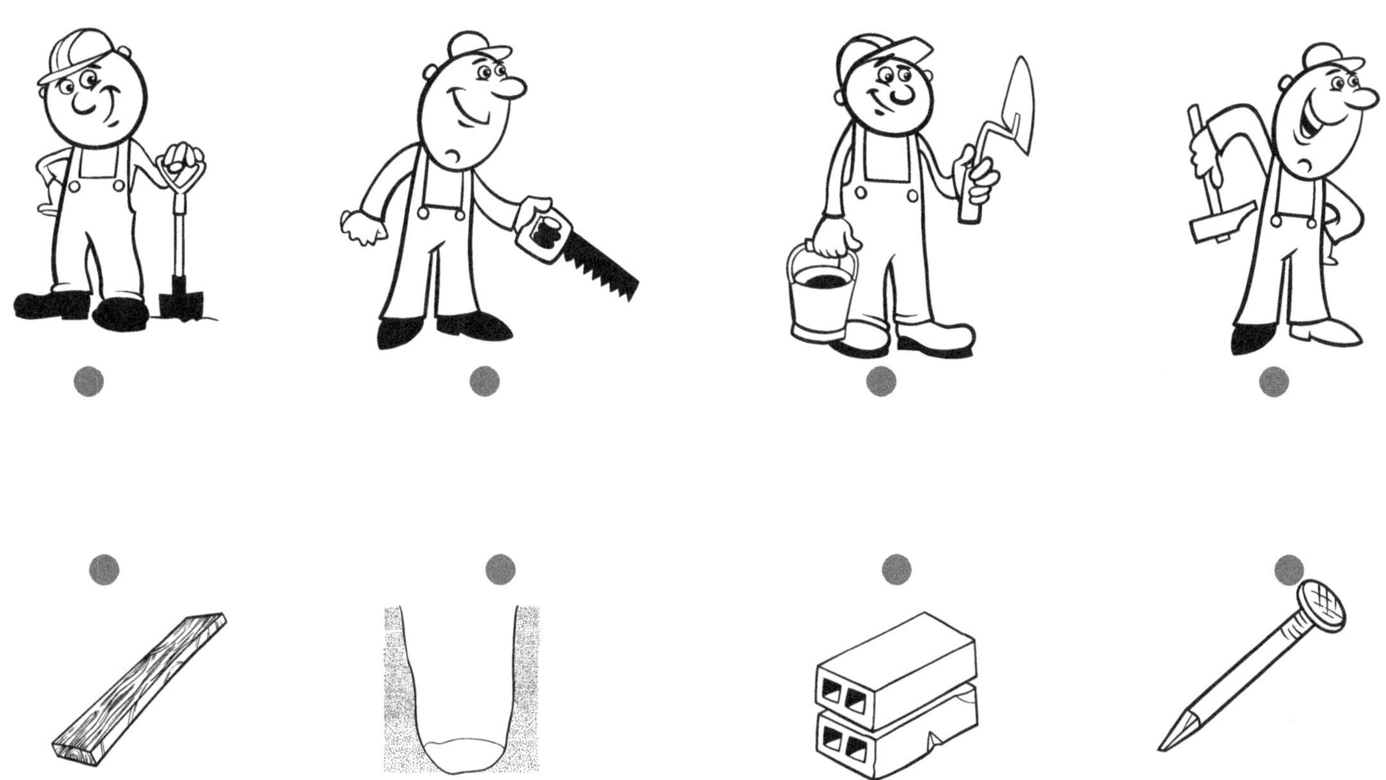

8. What would be useful in the kitchen?

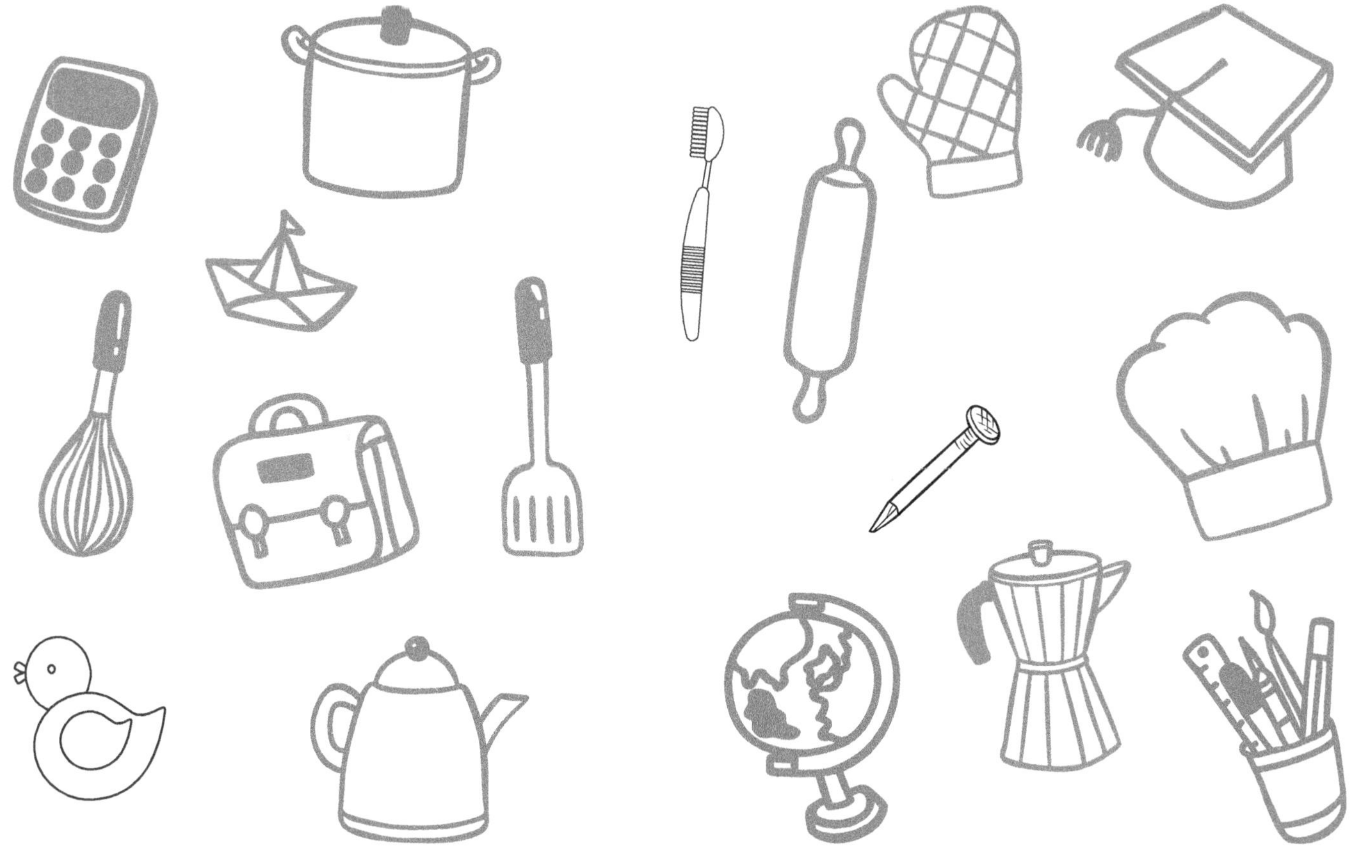

9. Write down what you see in the picture.

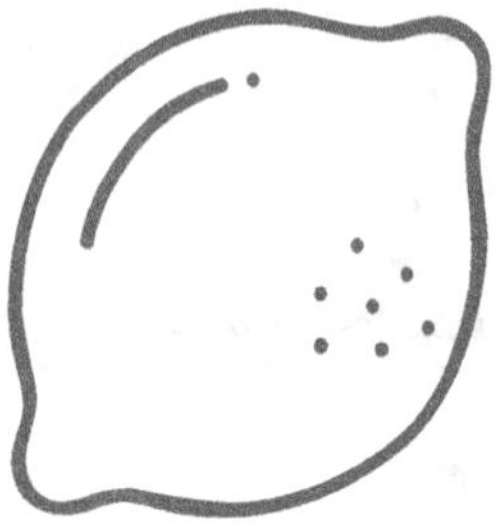

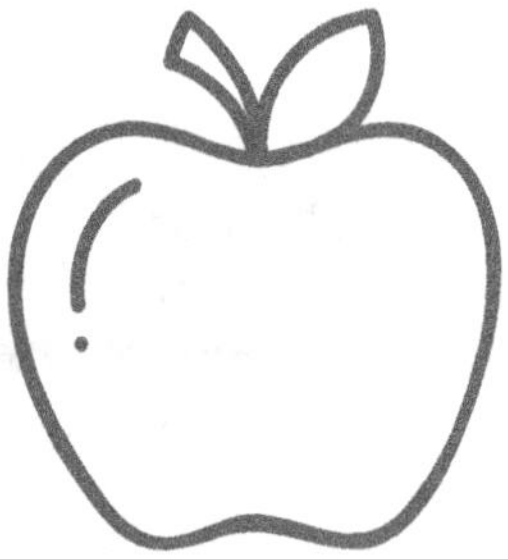

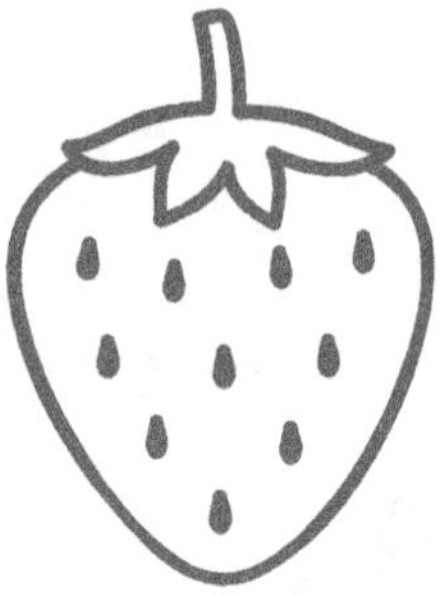

. . . .

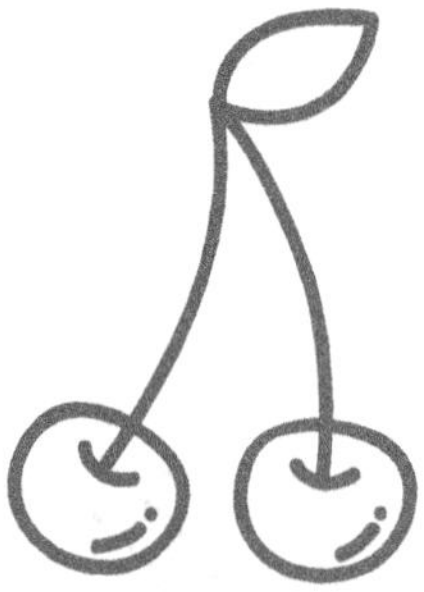

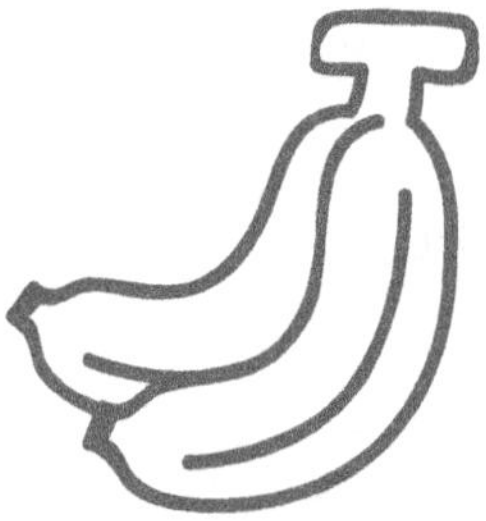

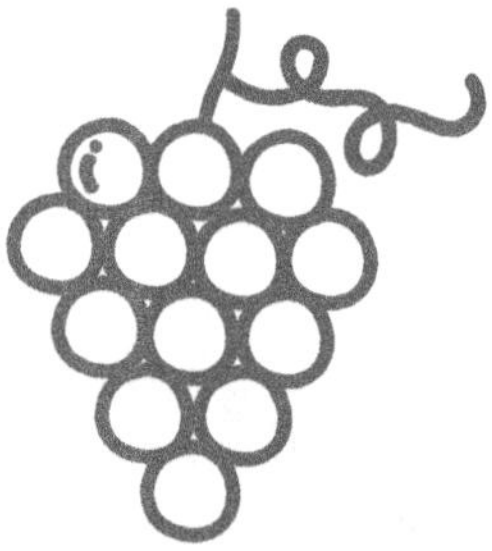

. . . .

10. List as many words as possible from the category
Months:

. . . .

. . . .

. . . .

. . . .

. . . .

. . . .

11. Counting game.

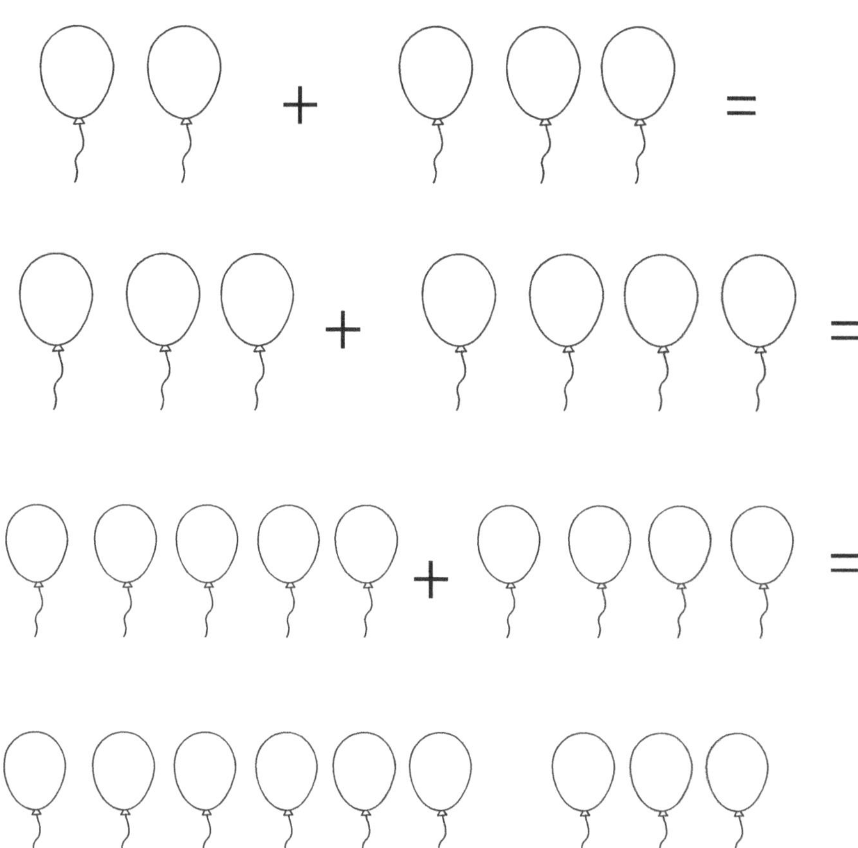

12. Match the shadow.

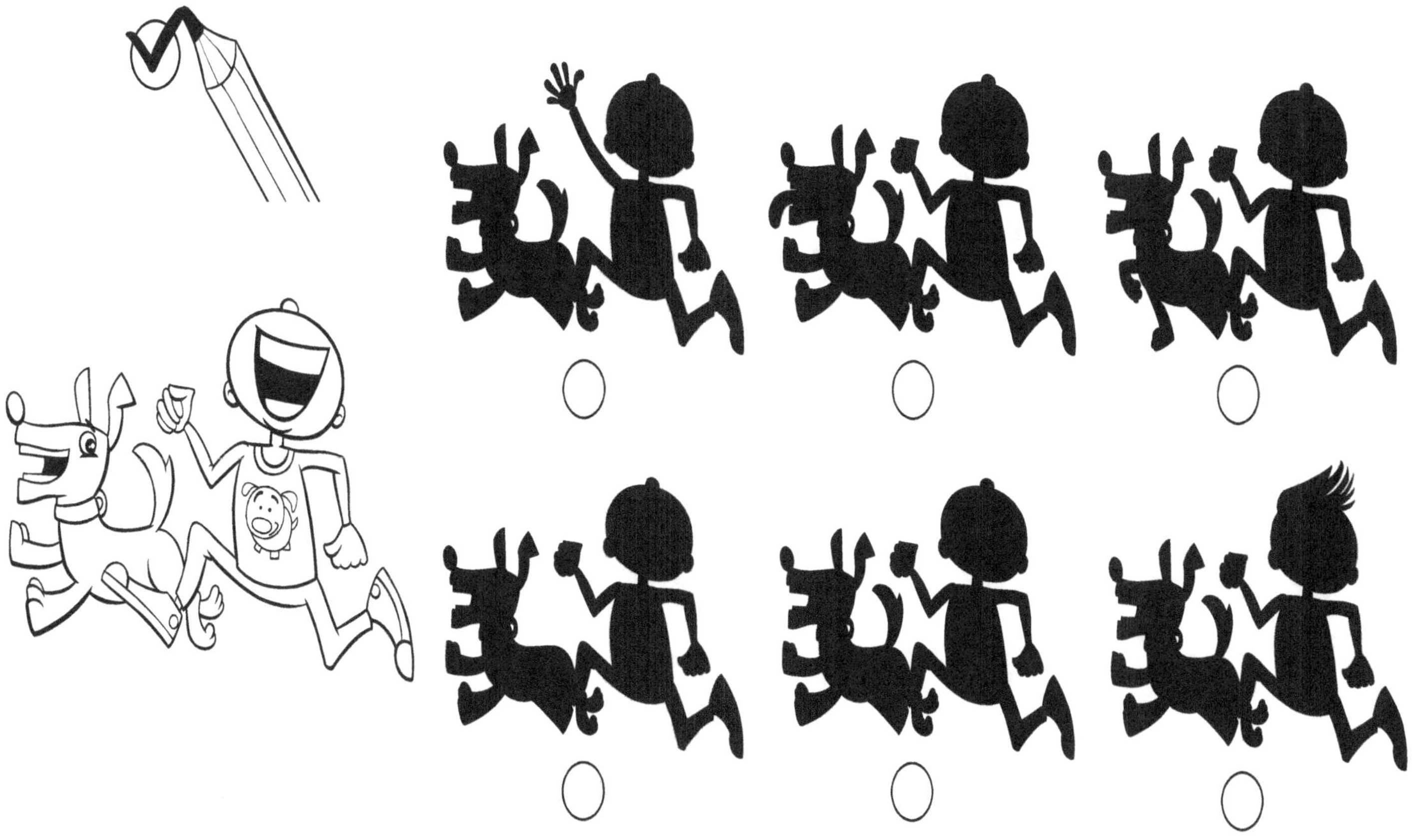

13. List as many words as possible from the category Fruit:

....

....

....

....

....

....

14. Dot to dot.

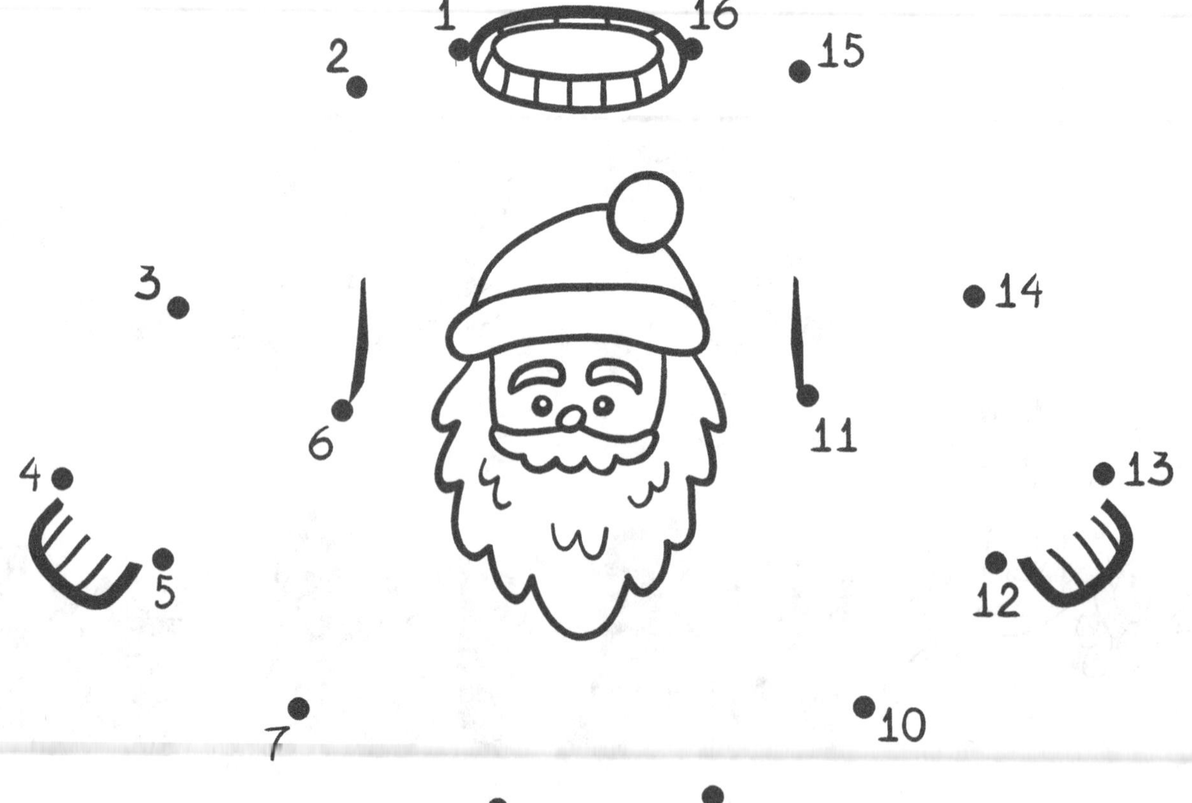

15. Write down what you see in the picture.

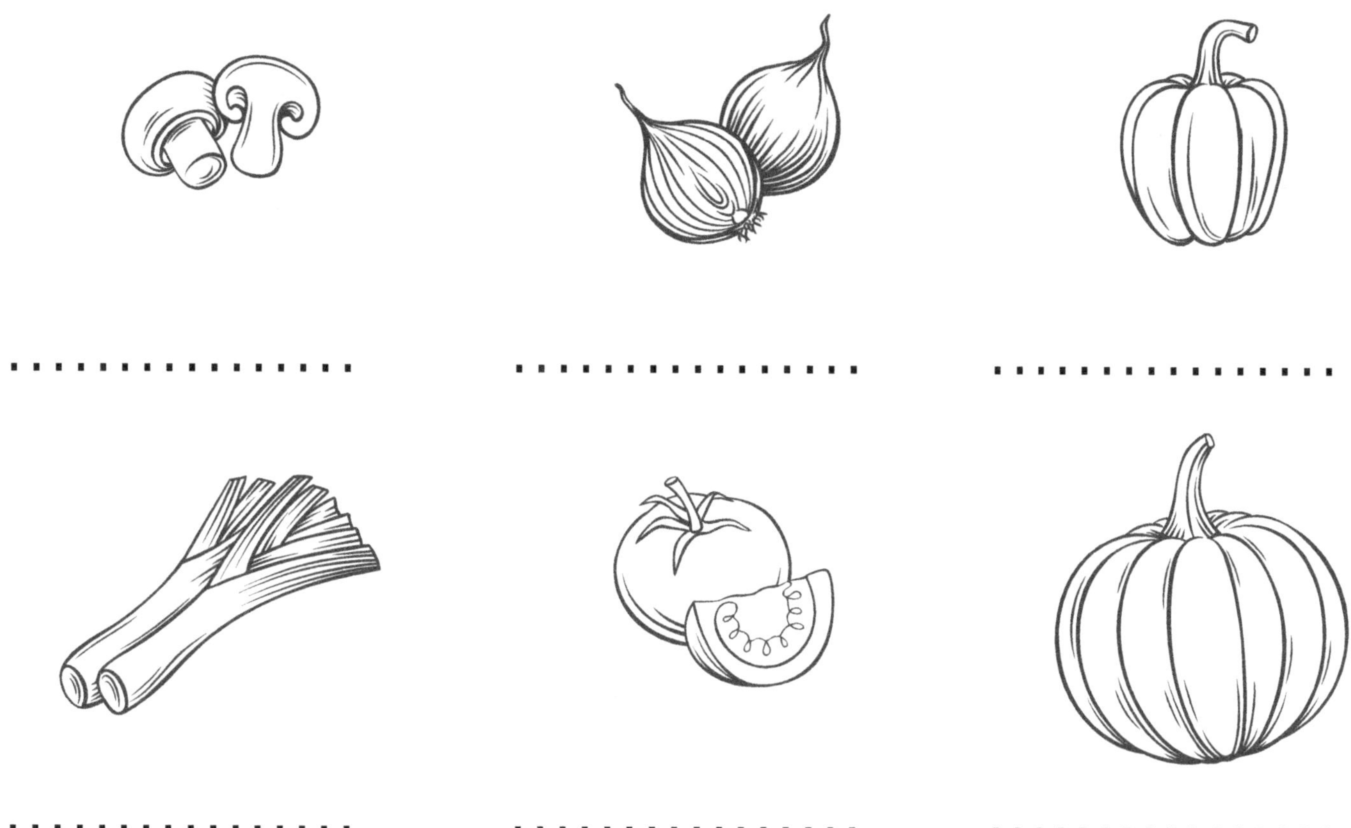

. . . .

. . . .

16. More or less?

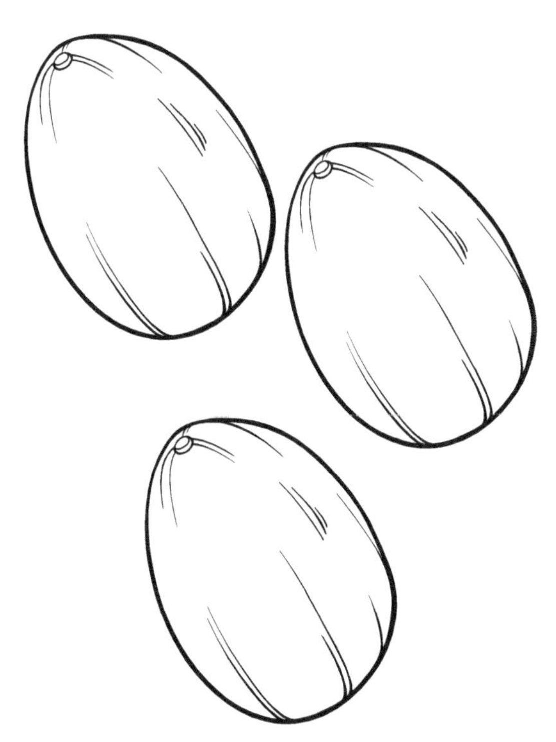

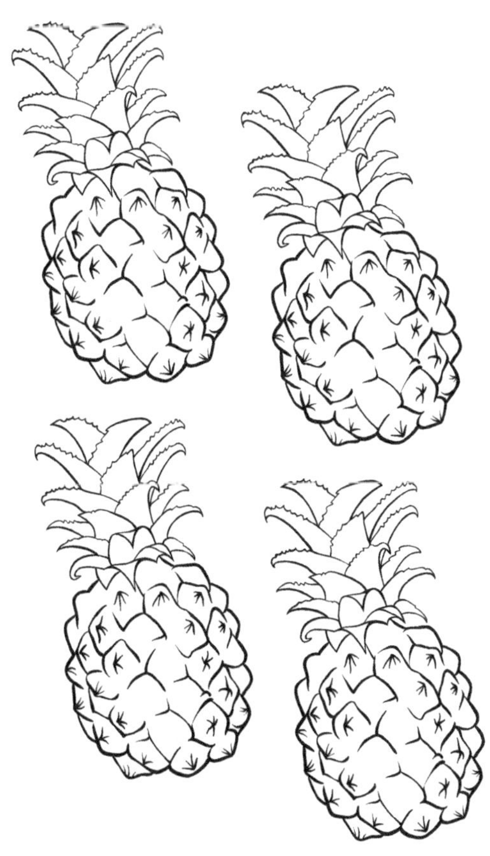

17. Word search.

P	S	W	I	N	D	Y	K
J	N	X	C	T	M	S	S
V	O	C	L	T	I	H	U
Z	W	I	O	F	S	P	N
L	R	C	U	R	T	V	N
B	A	E	D	O	P	B	Y
J	I	Y	Y	S	I	X	F
A	N	Q	W	T	R	J	R

ICE
MIST
RAIN
SNOW
SUNNY
FROST
CLOUDY
WINDY

18. Read and remember, cover with your hand and write from memory.

1 3 5 7	
11 21 31 41	

18. How many?

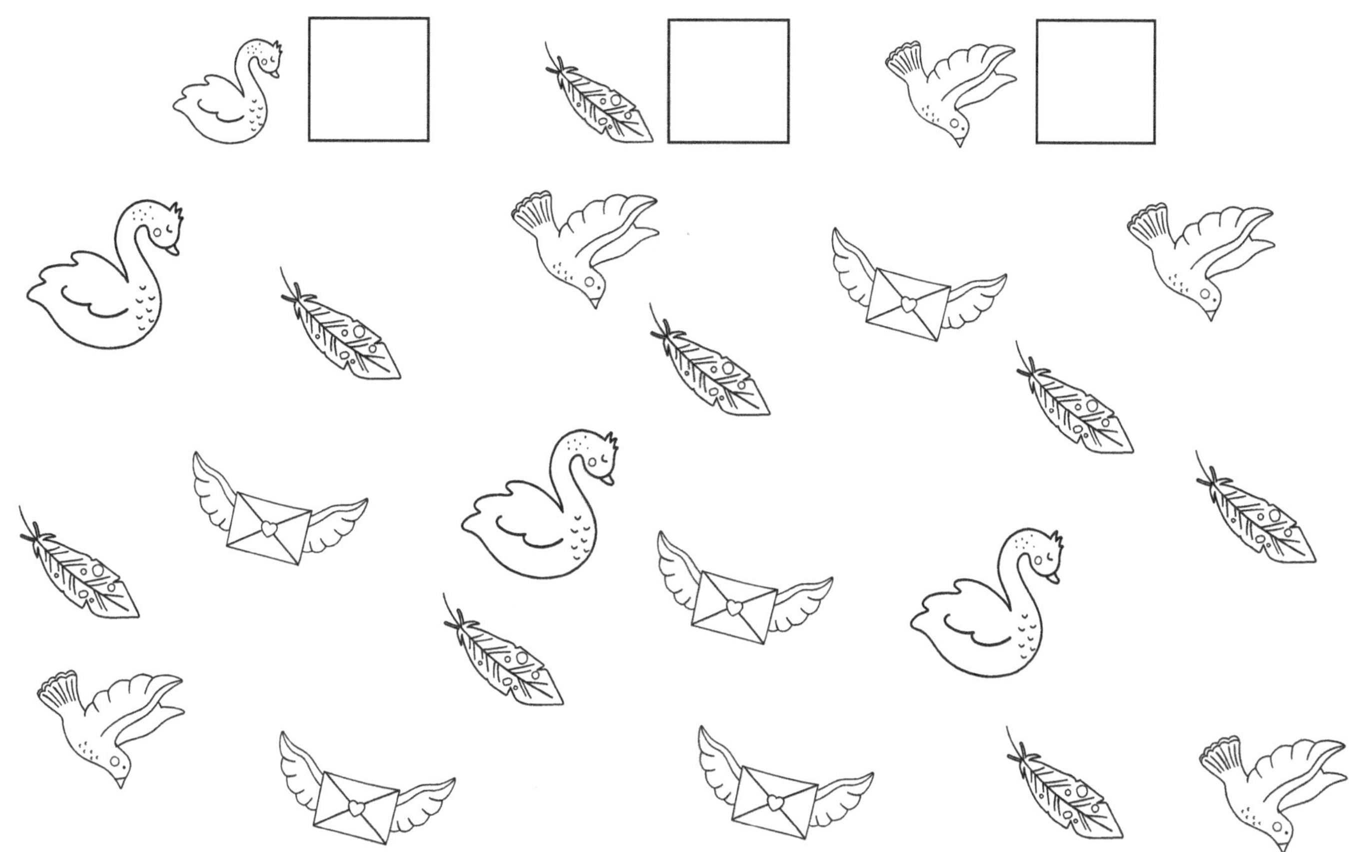

19. Counting game.

20. What does not fit?

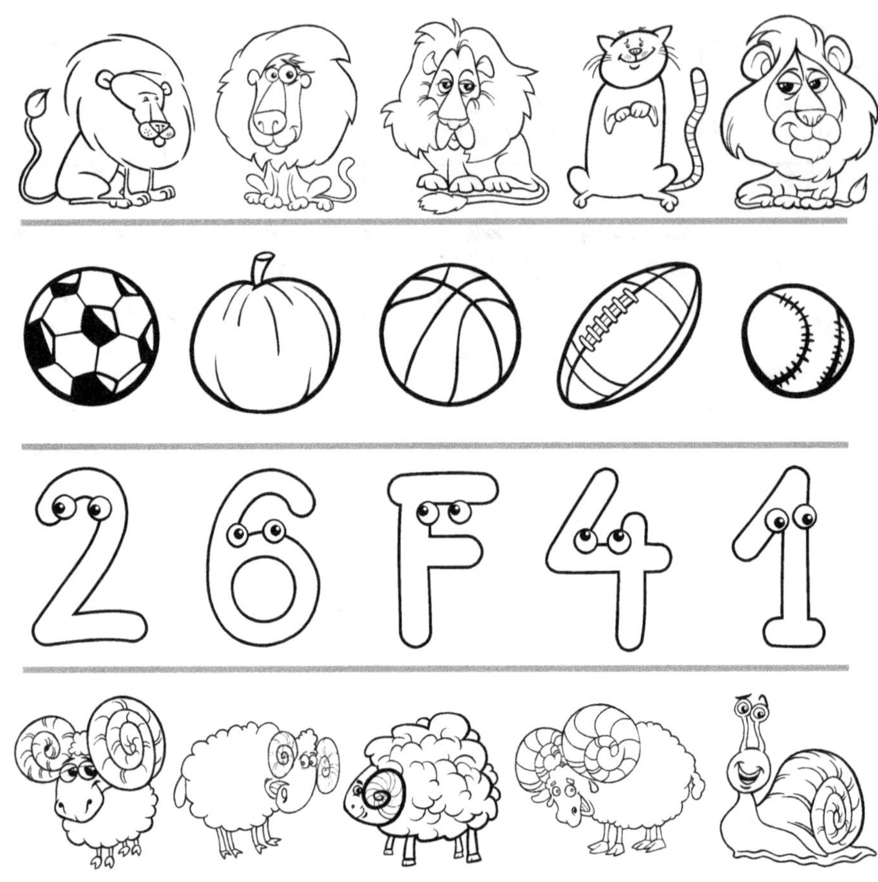

21. What is there that has no pair?

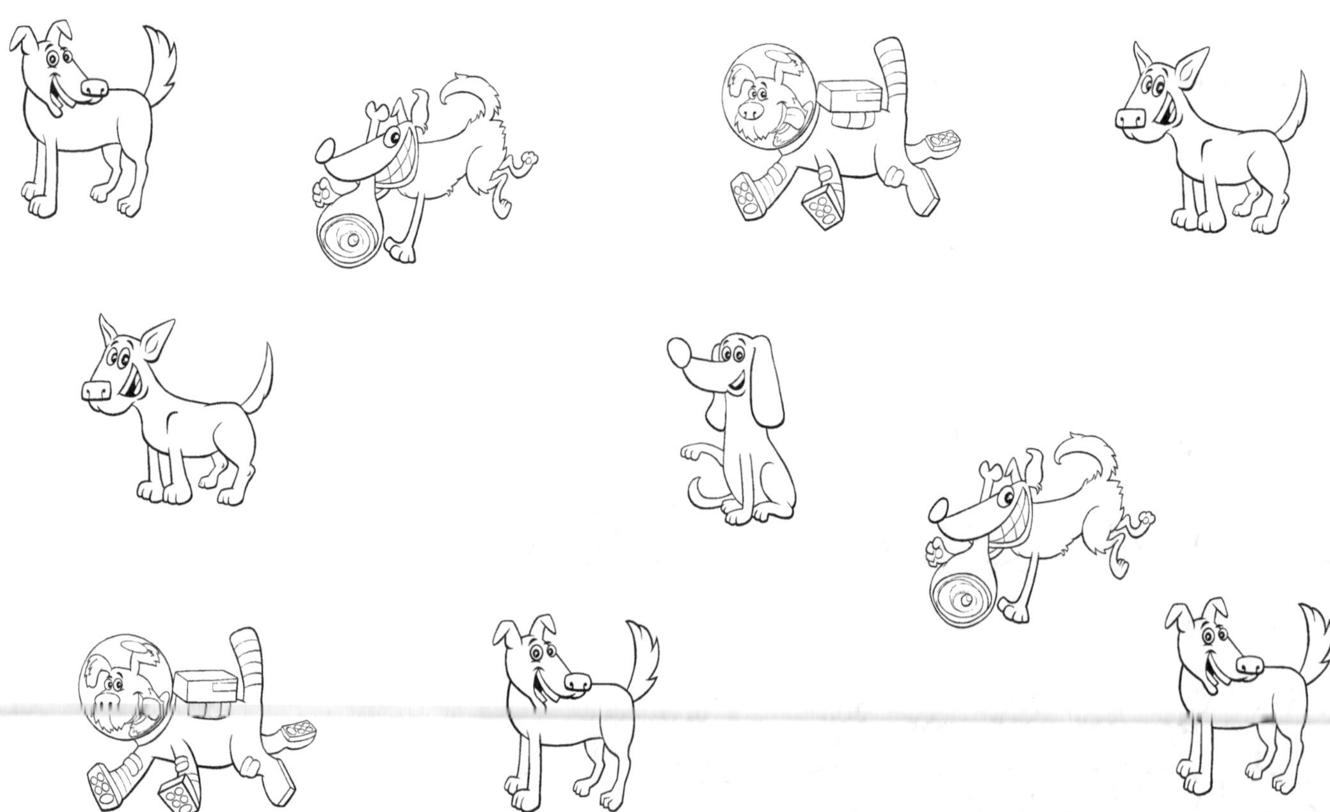

22. What would be useful in the bathroom?

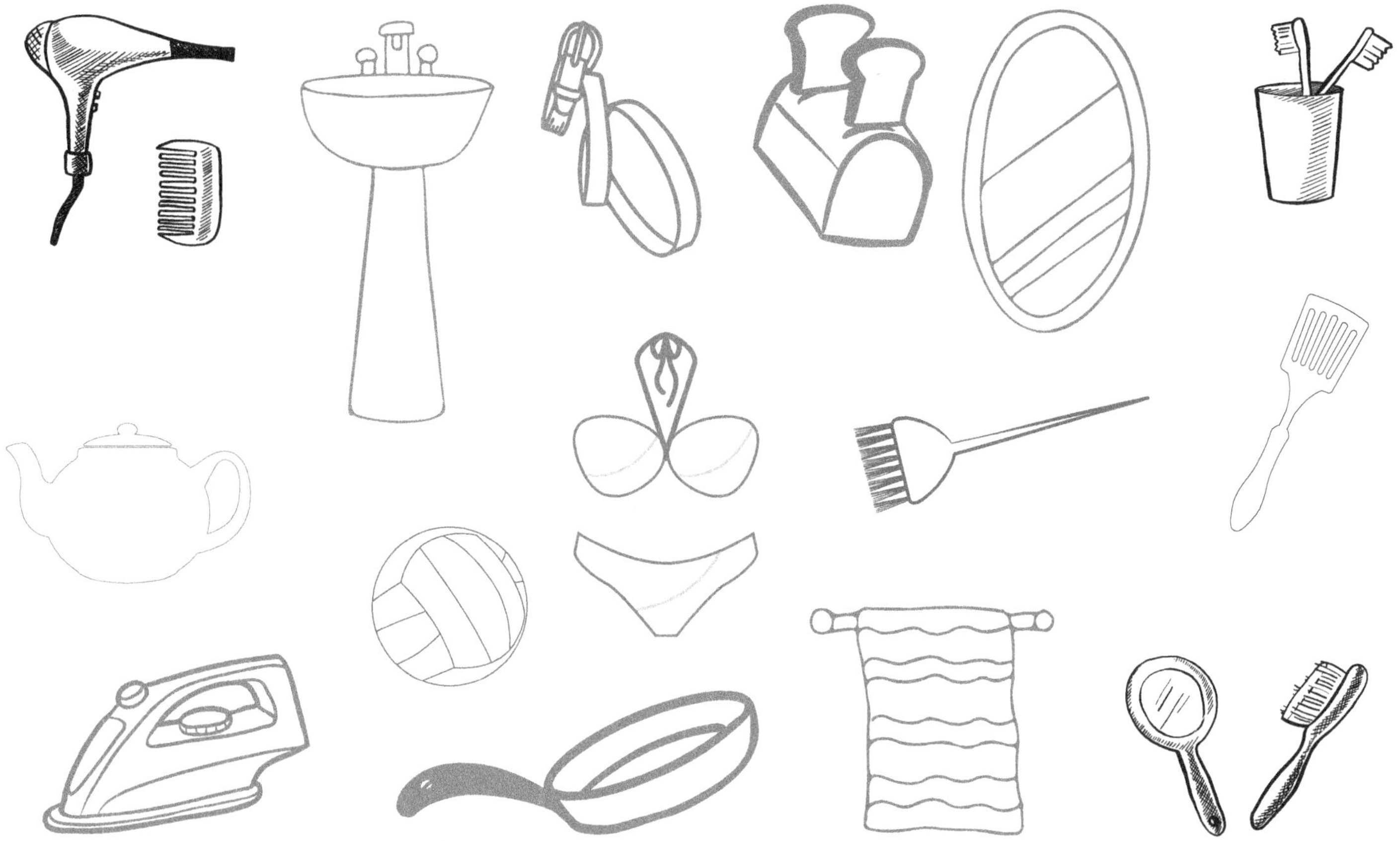

23. Number from the smallest to the largest.

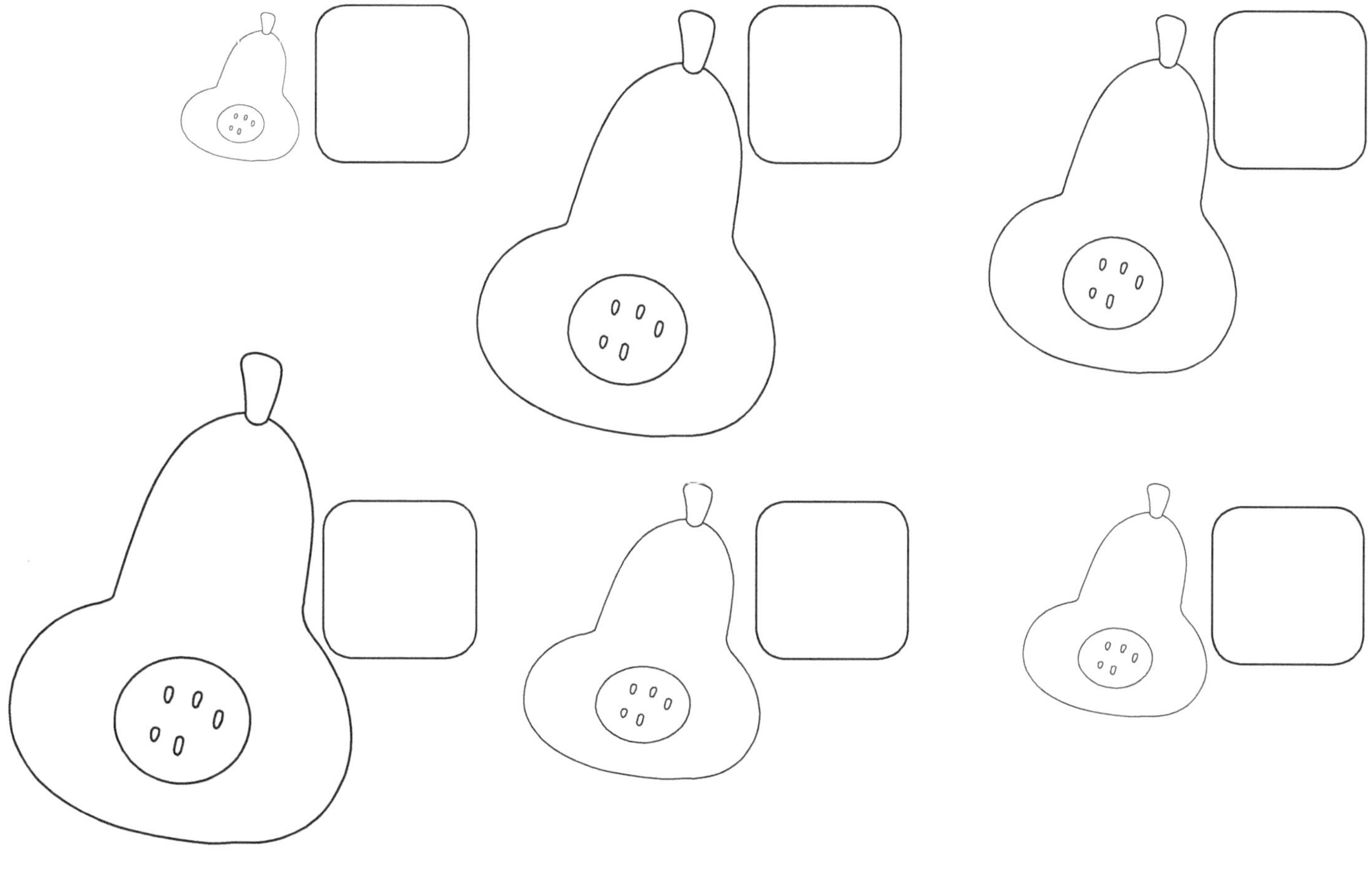

24. Read and remember, cover with your hand and write from memory.

22 33 44 55	
45 55 65 75	

25. Find 5 differences.

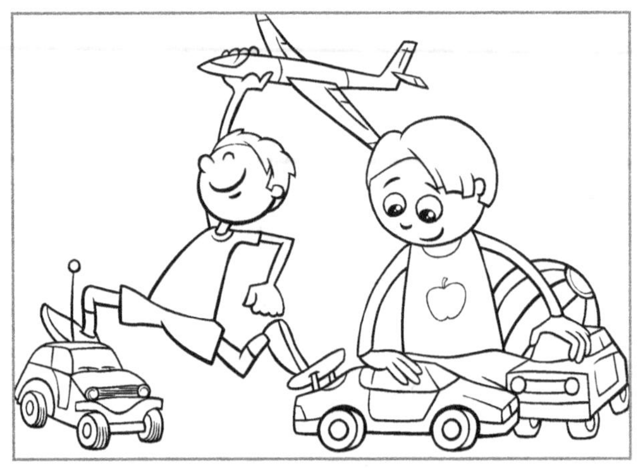

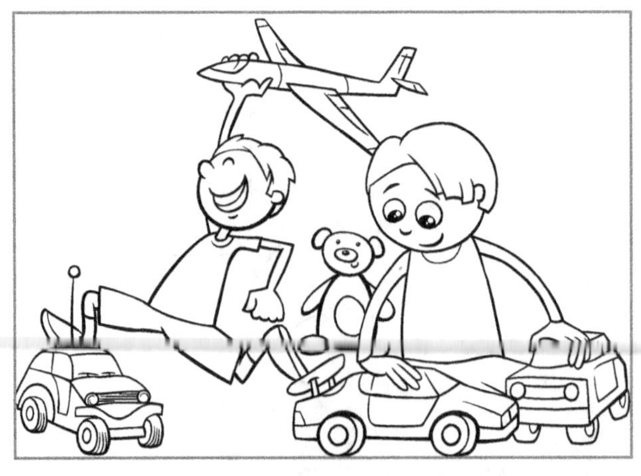

26.Dot to dot.

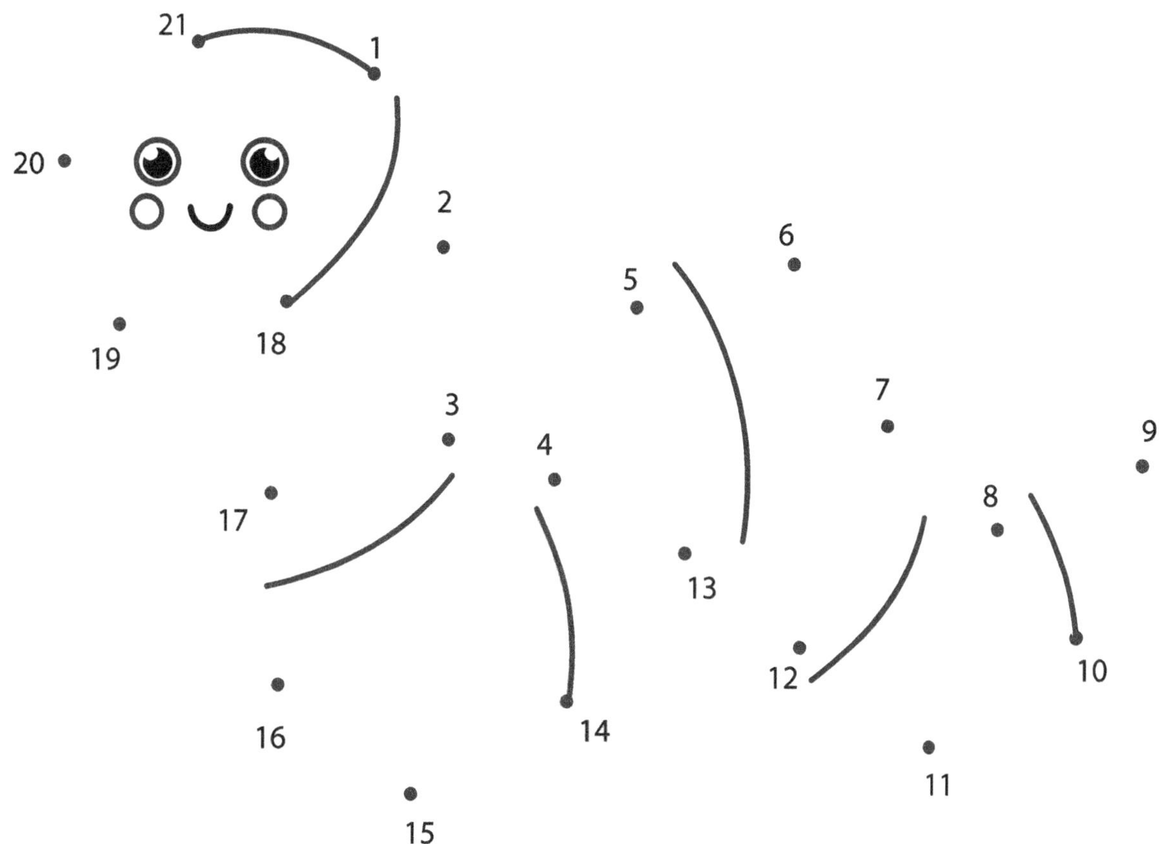

27. What would be useful for a student at school?

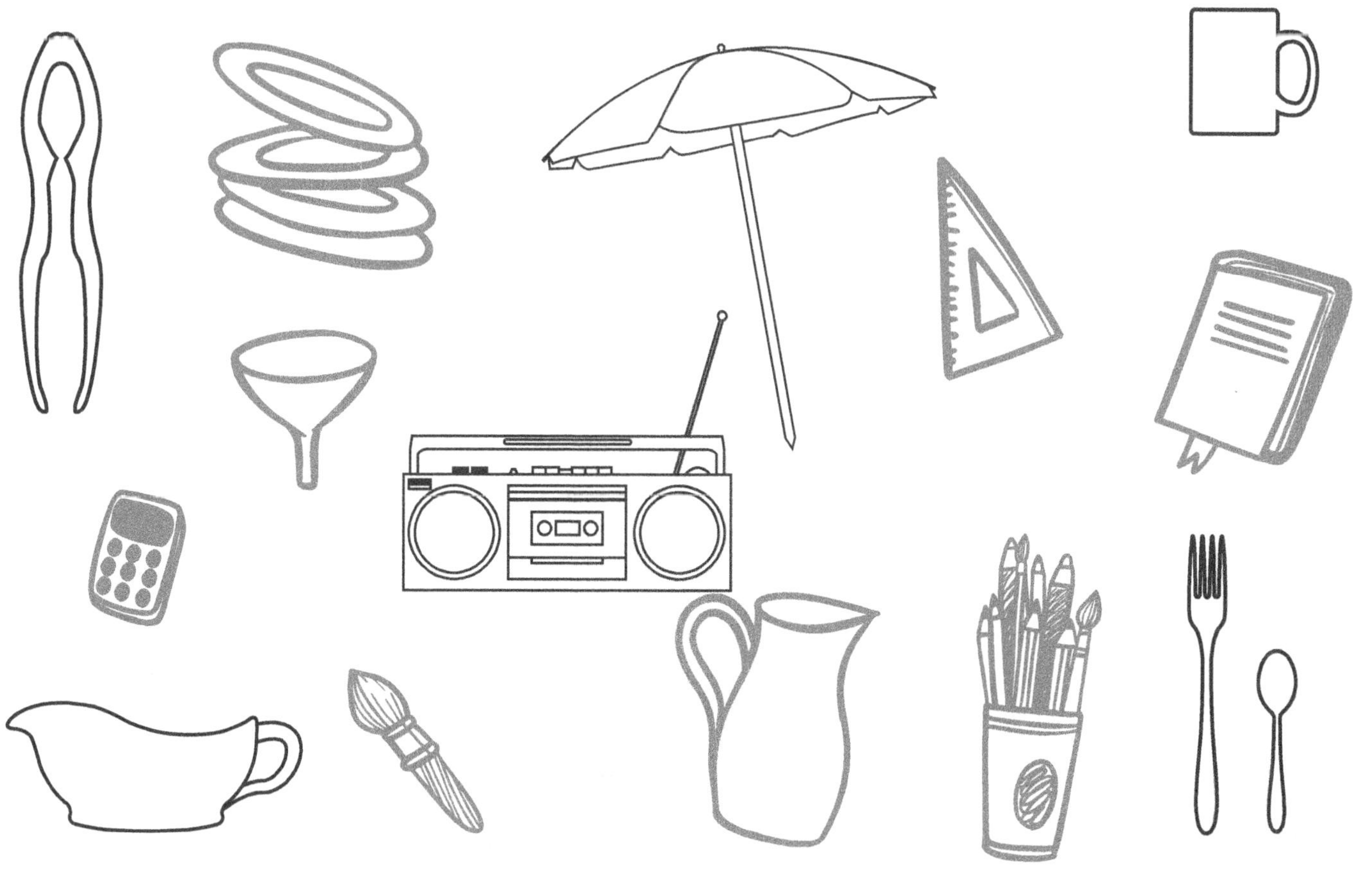

28. What does not fit?

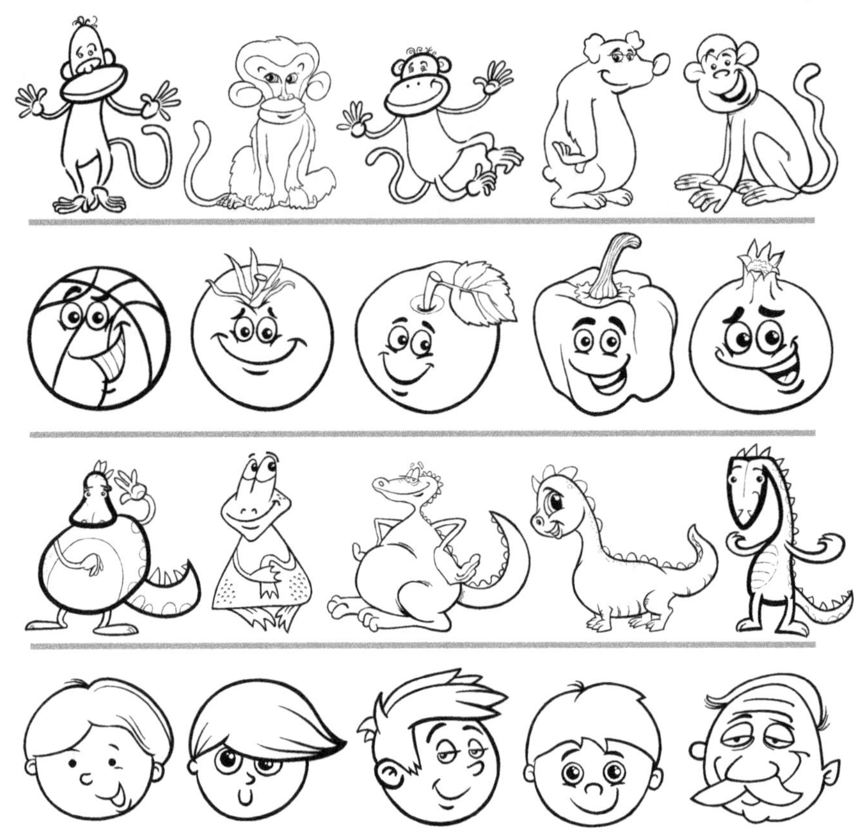

29. Match pairs.

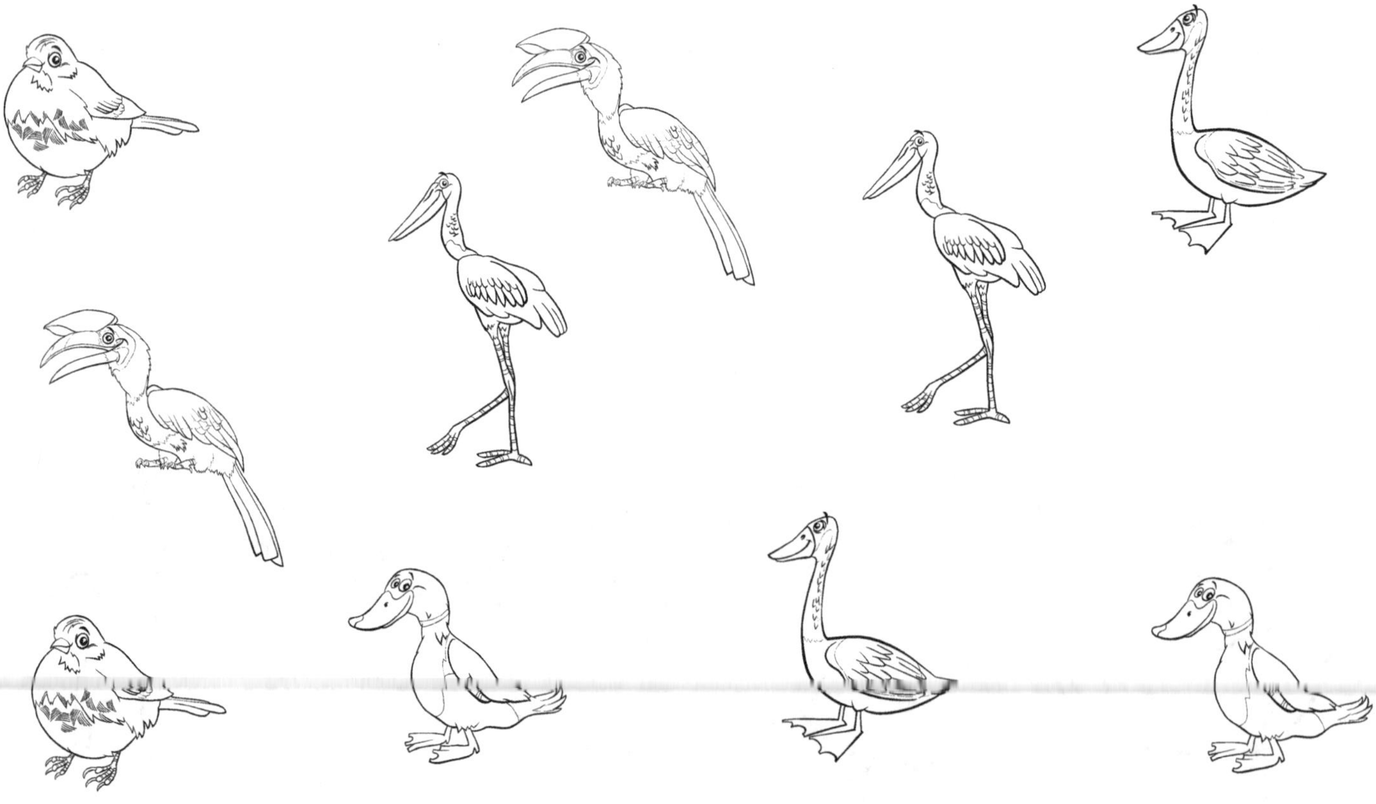

30. Write down what you see in the picture.

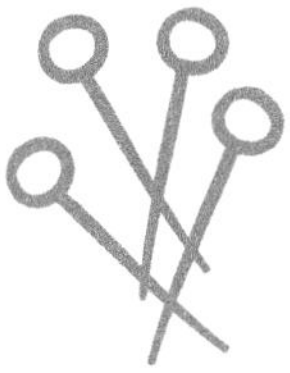

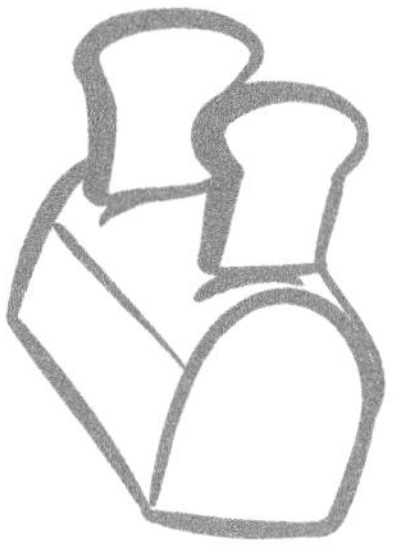

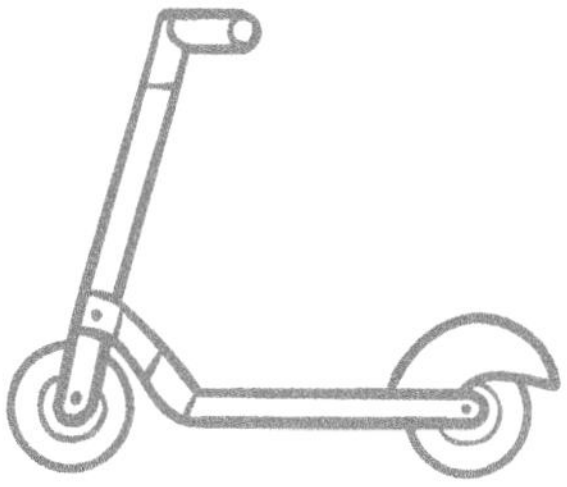

. . . .

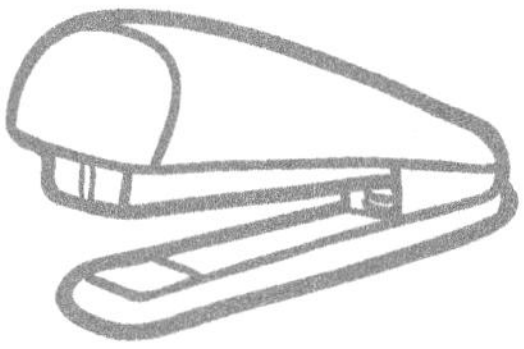

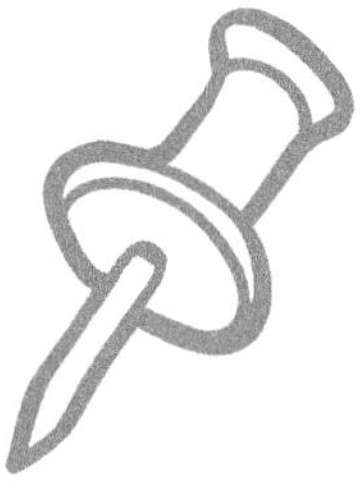

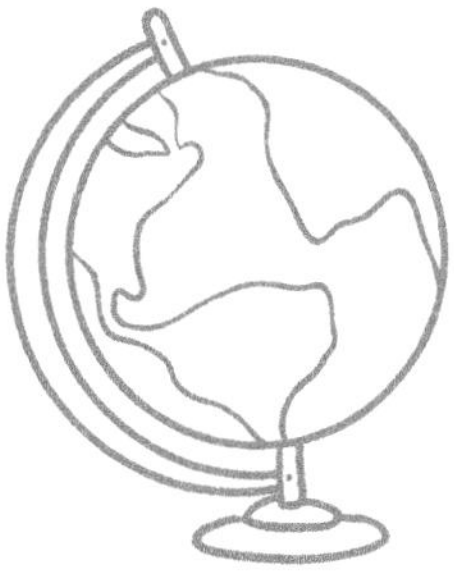

. . . .

31. List as many words as possible from the category
Vegetables:

. . . .

. . . .

. . . .

. . . .

. . . .

. . . .

32. Counting game.

 × **2** =

× **2** =

× **3** =

× **2** =

33. Write down what you see in the picture.

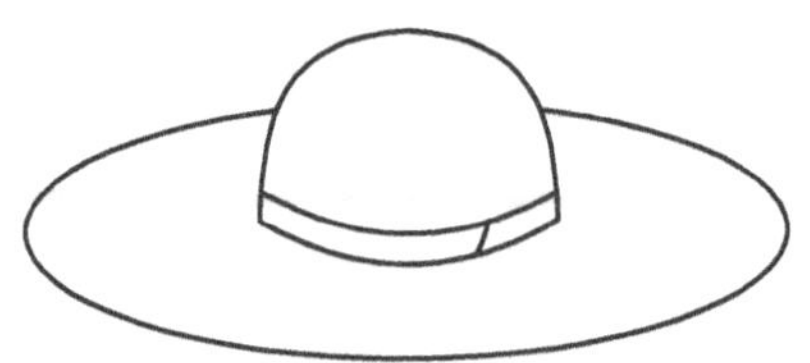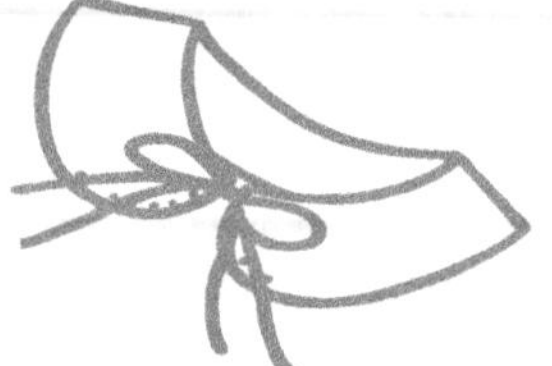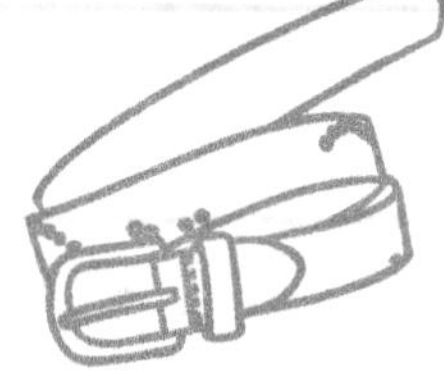

. . . .

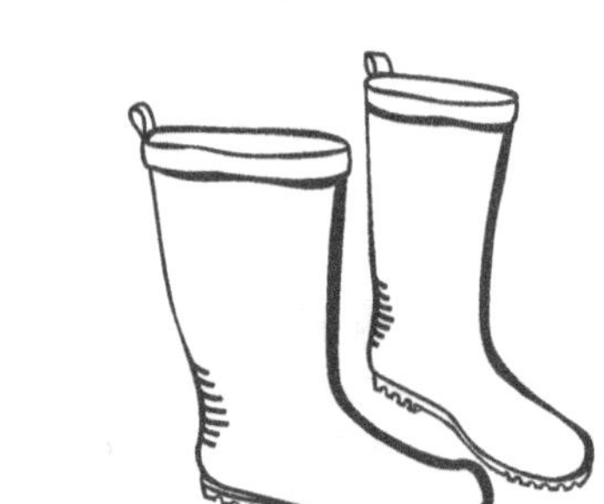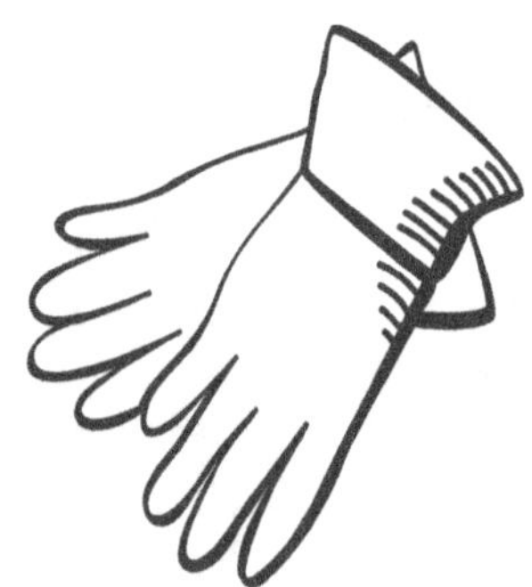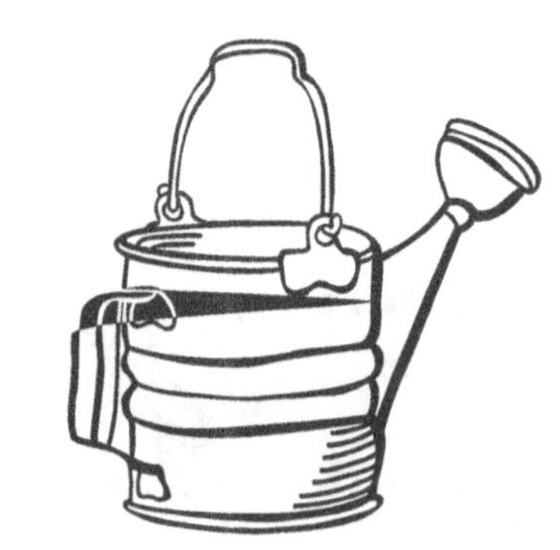

. . . .

34. How many?

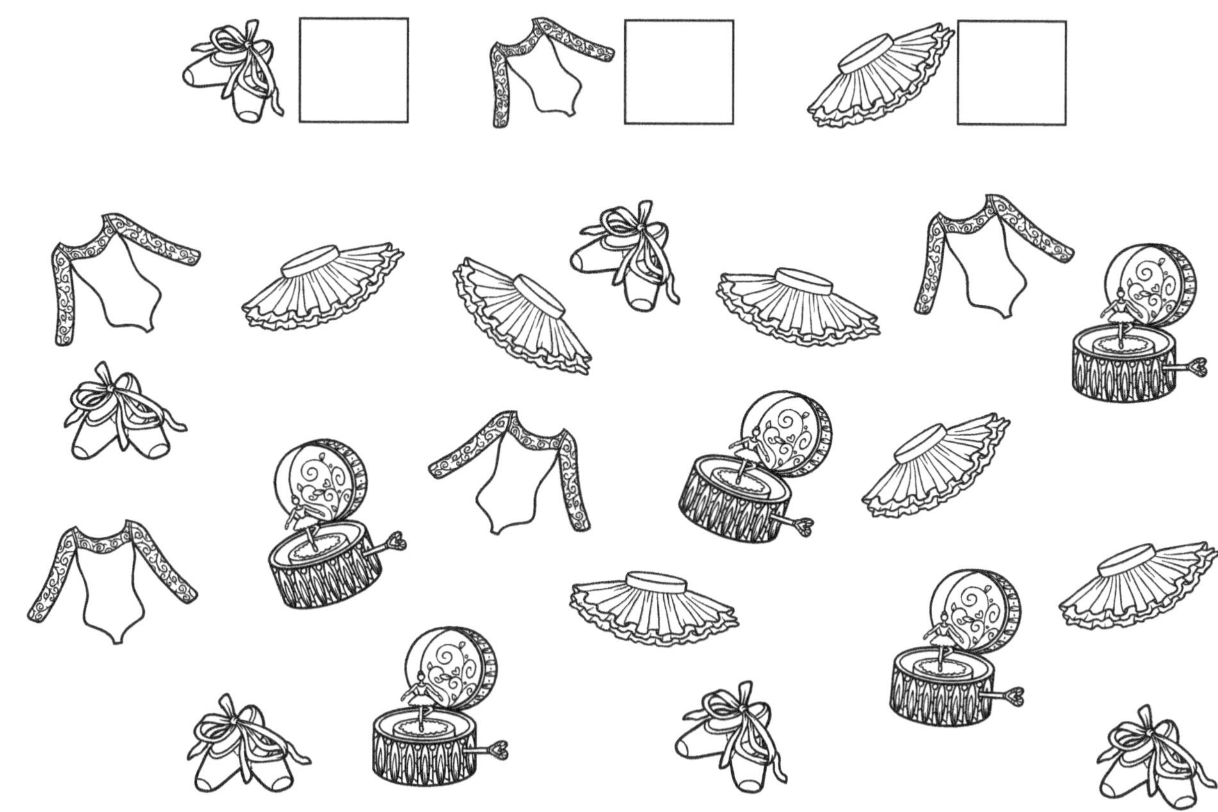

35. More or less?

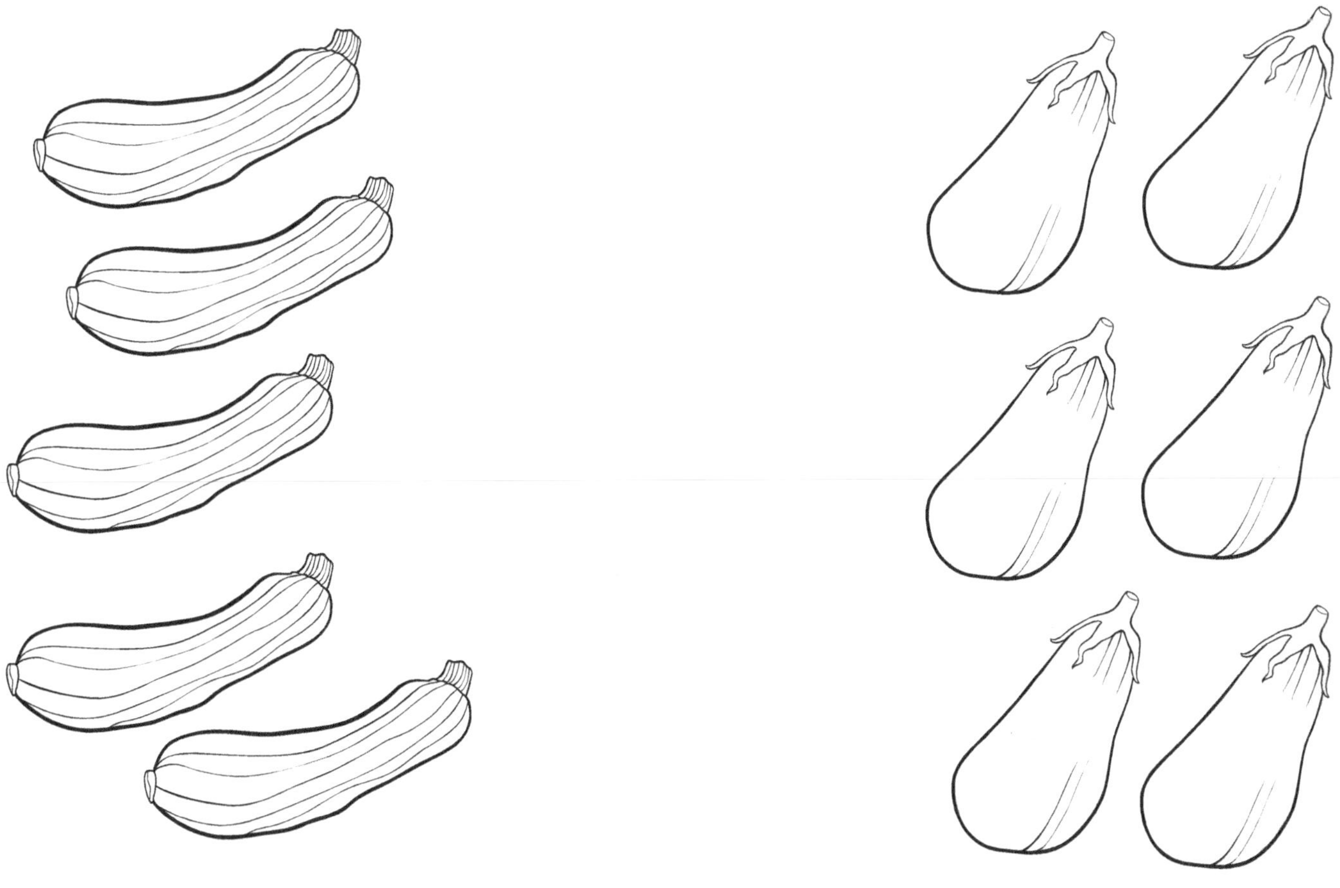

36. What is there that has no pair?

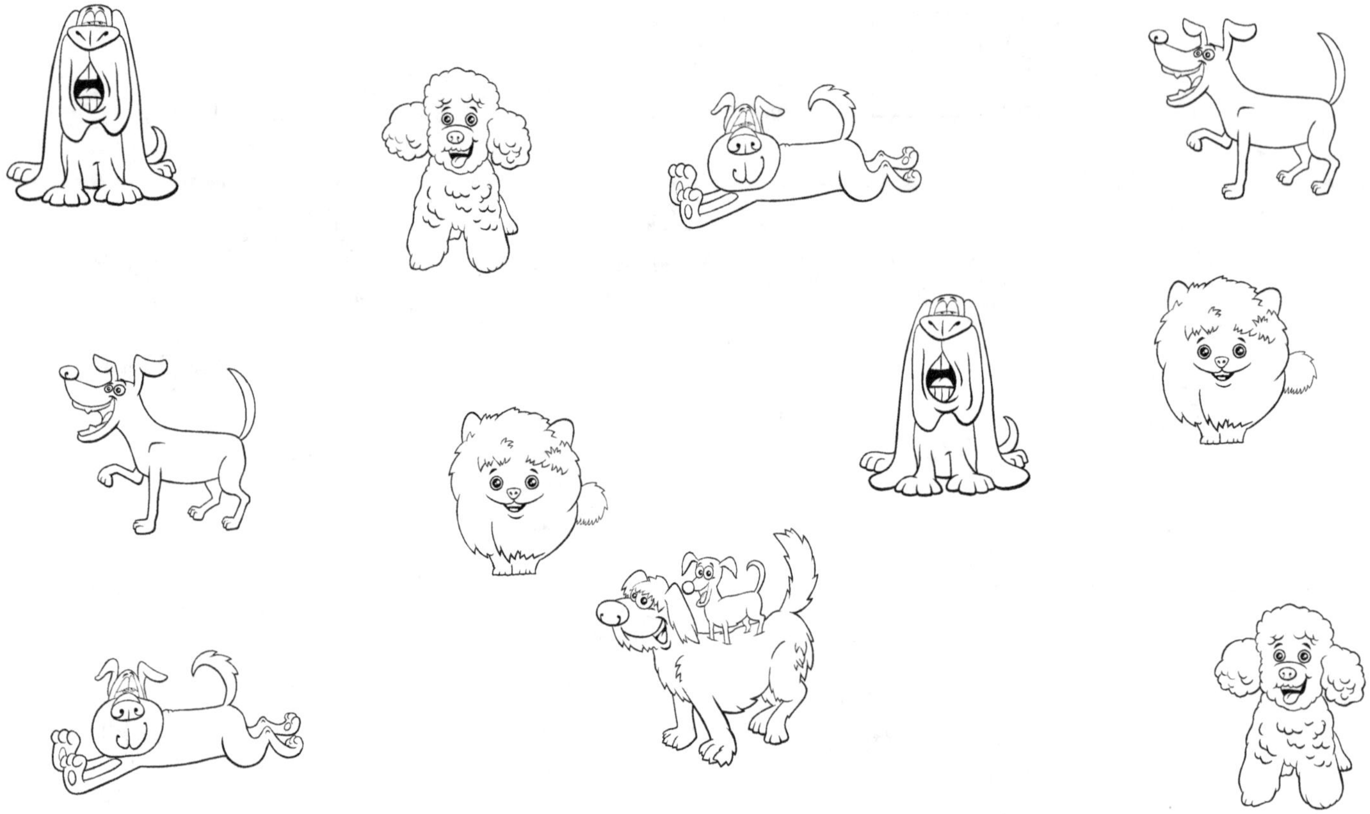

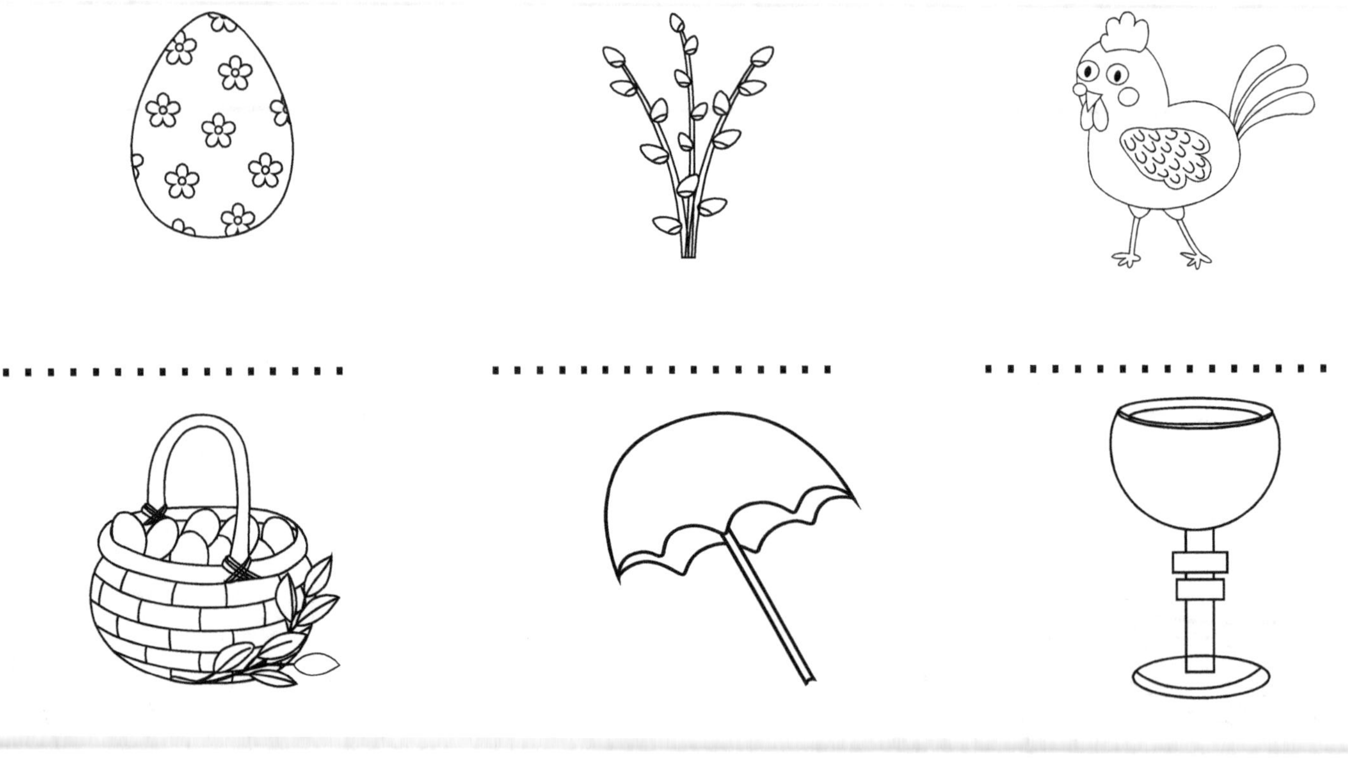

37. Write down what you see in the picture.

38. Match words with the correct pictures.

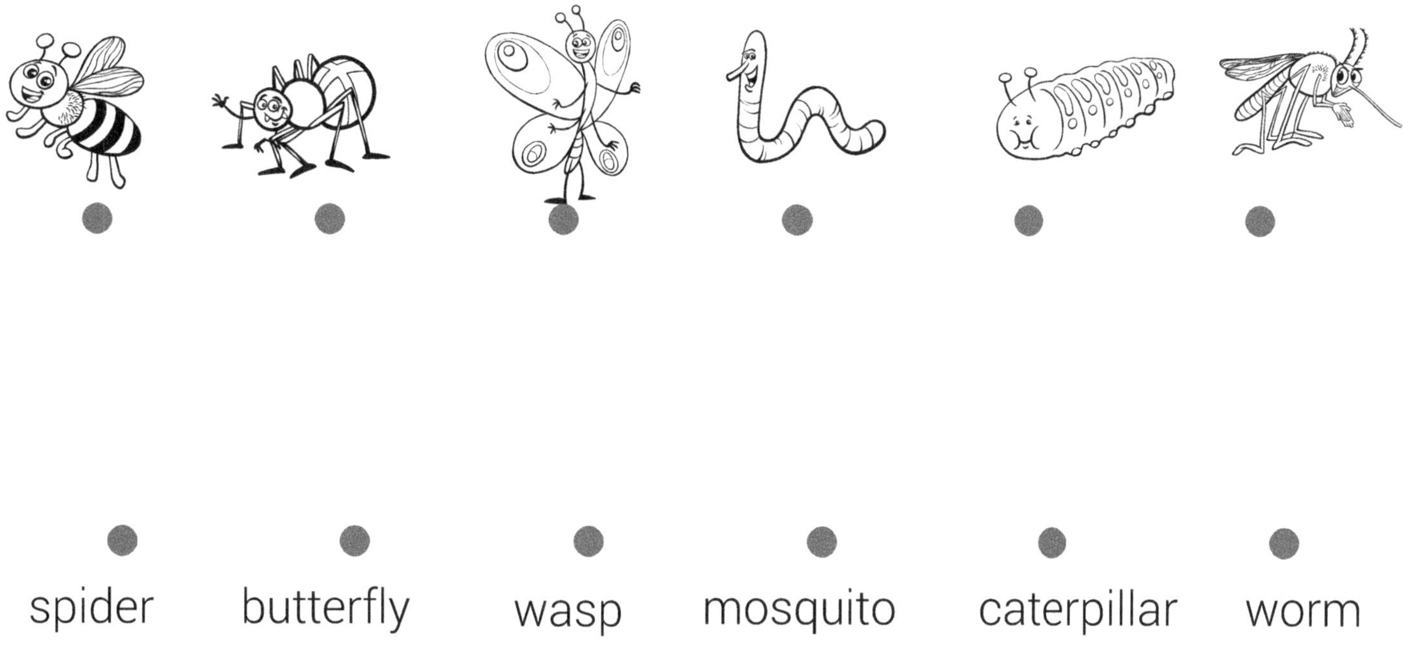

spider   butterfly   wasp   mosquito   caterpillar   worm

39. Read and remember, cover with your hand and write from memory.

kiwi grapefruit coconut	
strawberry blackberry blueberry	

40. Write the numbers using words.

4-..

6-..

7-..

9-..

10-..

11-..

13-..

41. Dot to dot.

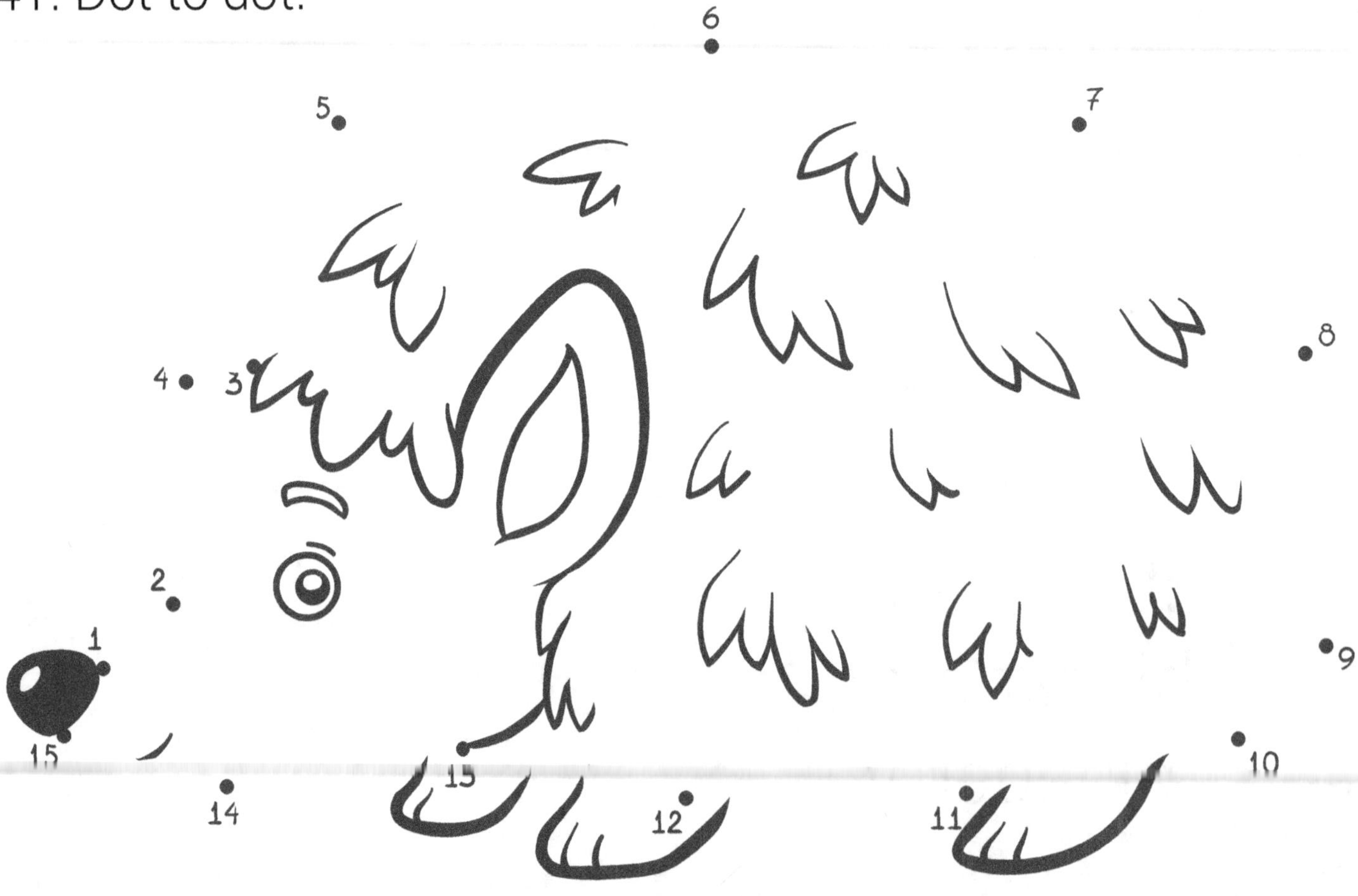

42. Matching game.

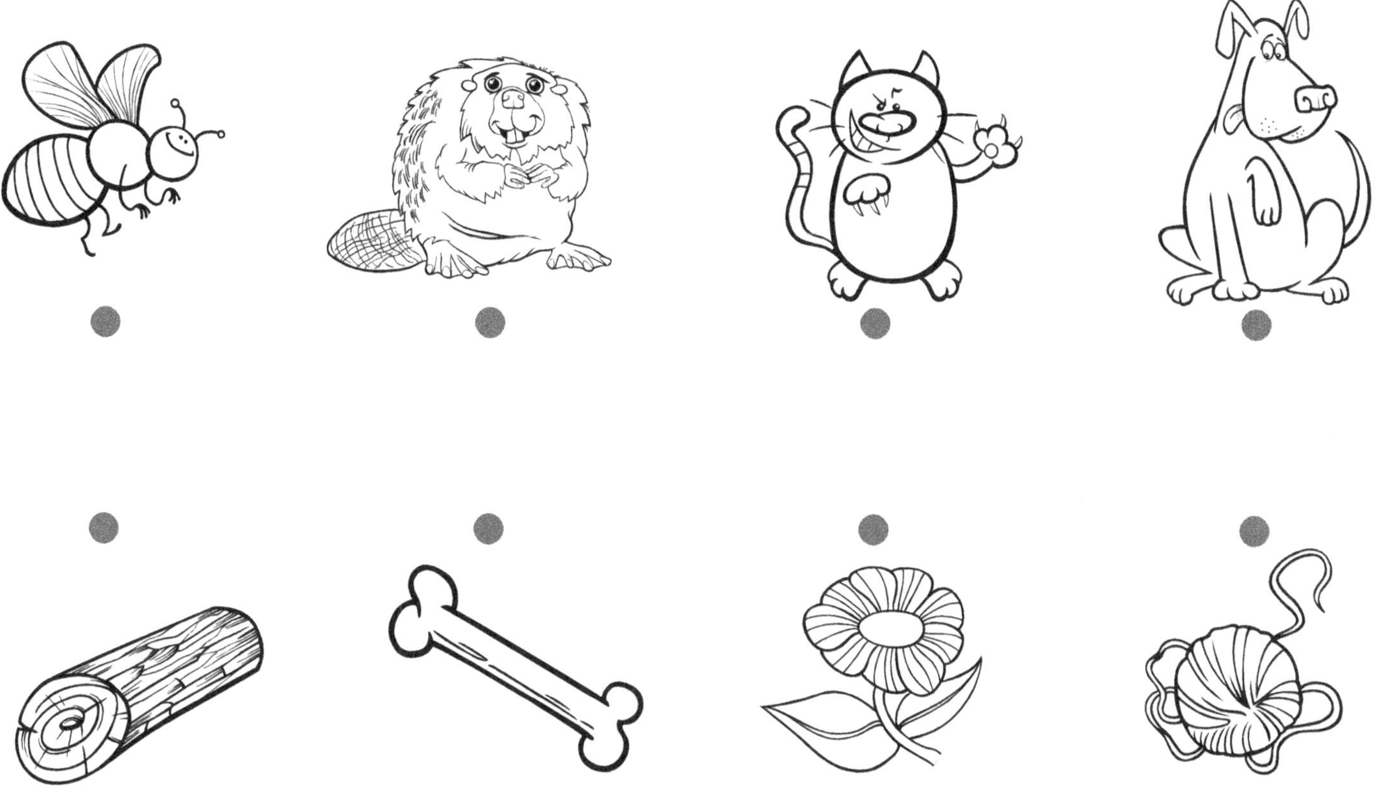

43. What is there that has no pair?

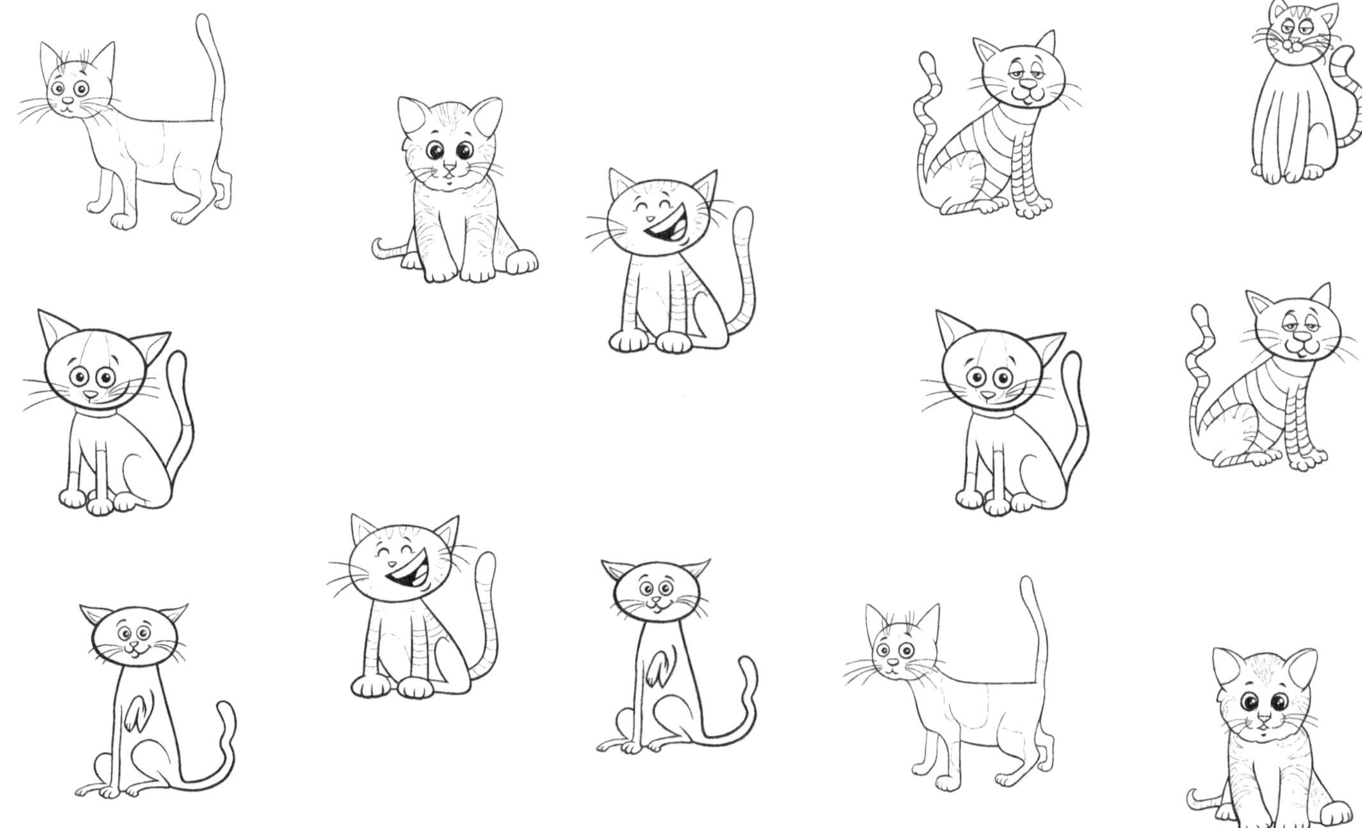

44. Mark insects with one color and birds with a different one.

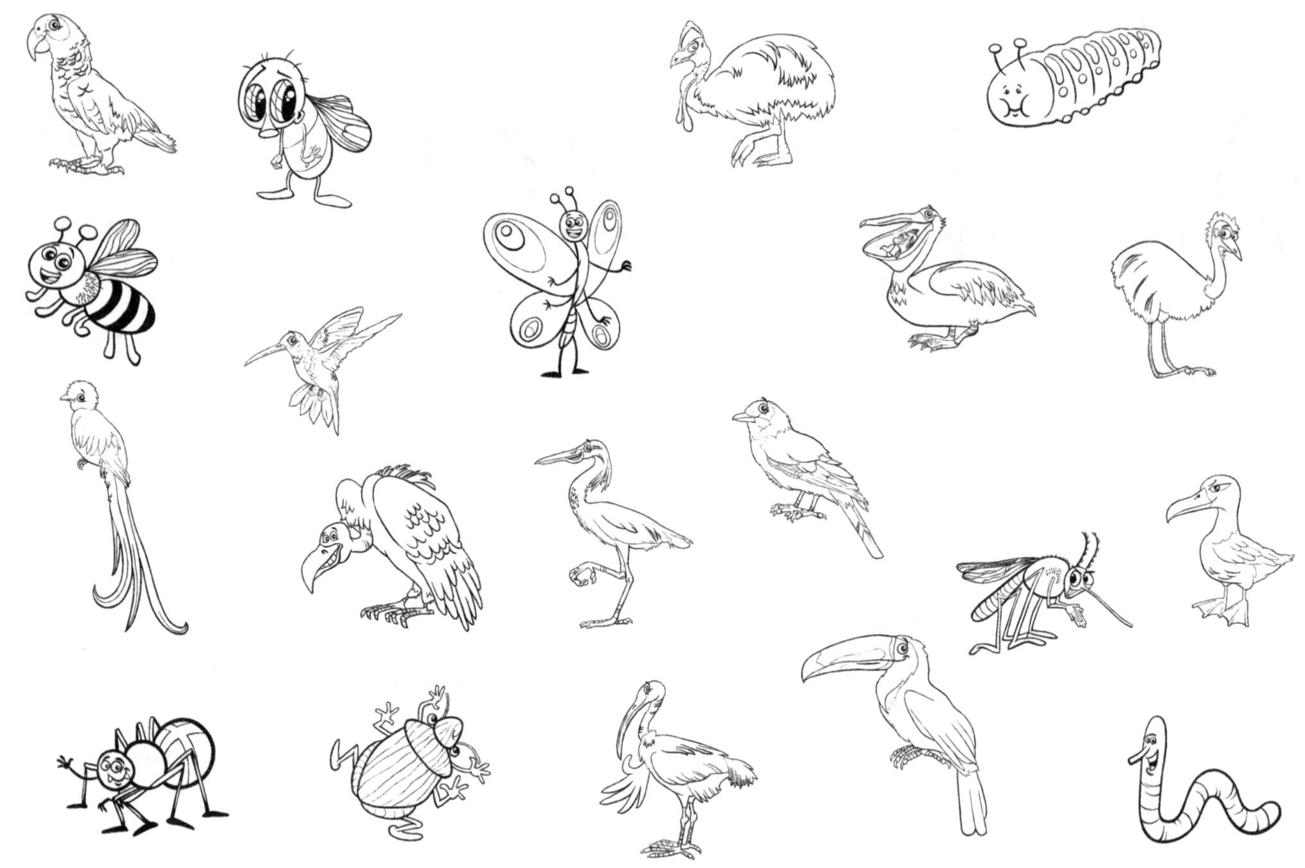

45. Counting game.

$$\bigcirc\bigcirc\bigcirc \times 2 =$$

$$\times 2 =$$

$$\times 3 =$$

$$\times 2 =$$

46. What does not fit?

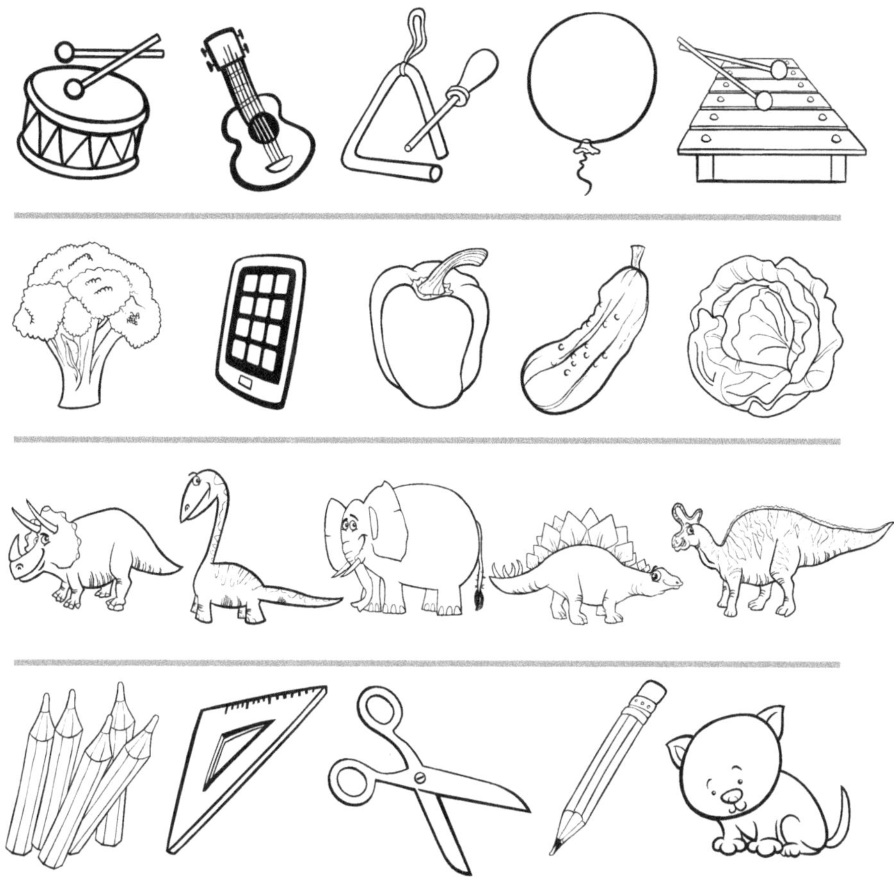

47. List as many words as possible from the category
Toys:

....

....

....

....

....

....

48. More or less?

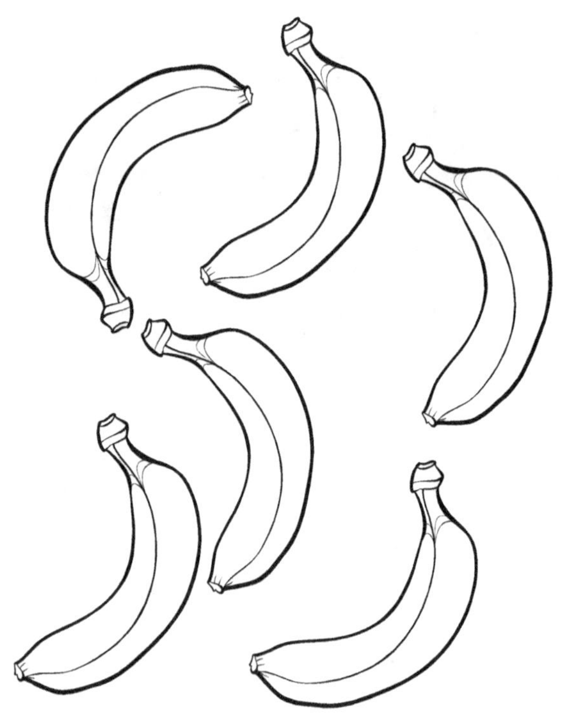 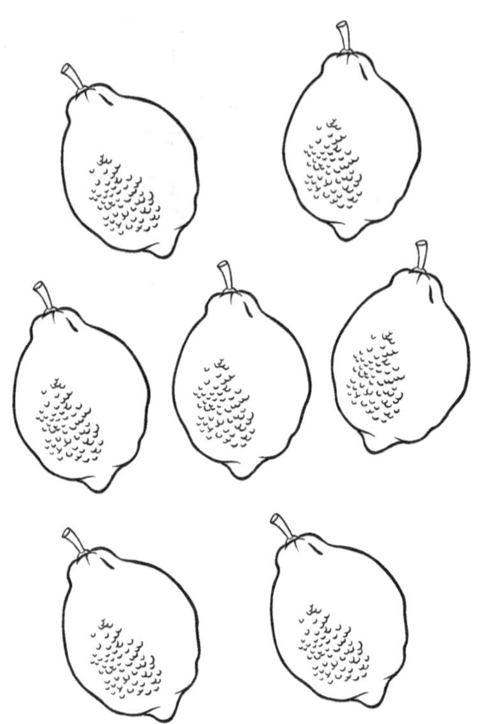

49. Write down what you see in the picture.

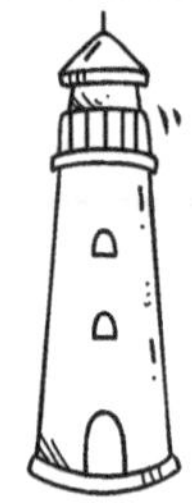  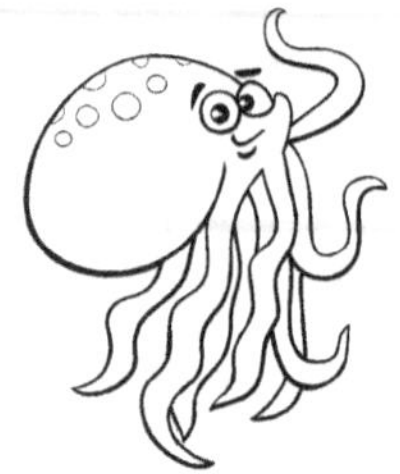

. . . .

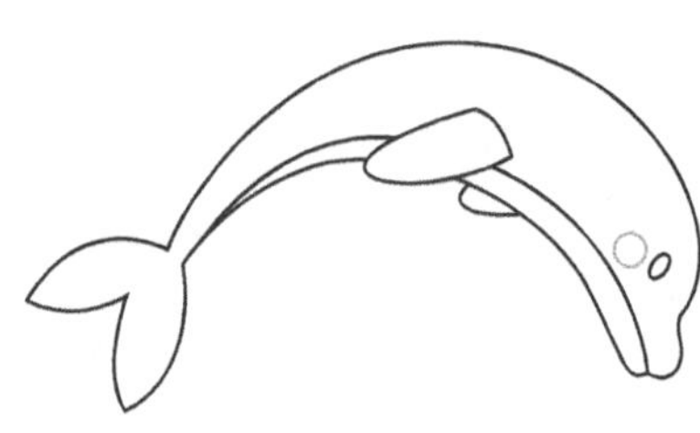 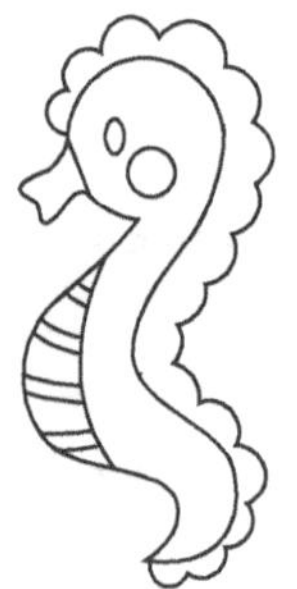 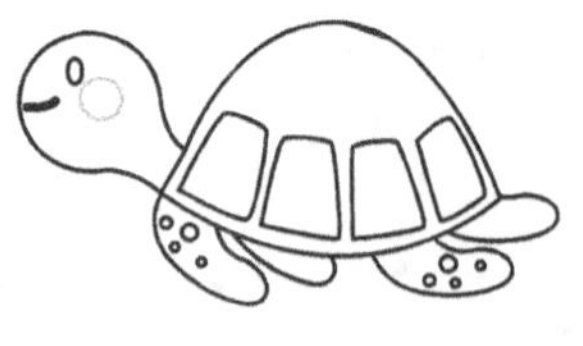

. . . .

50. How many?

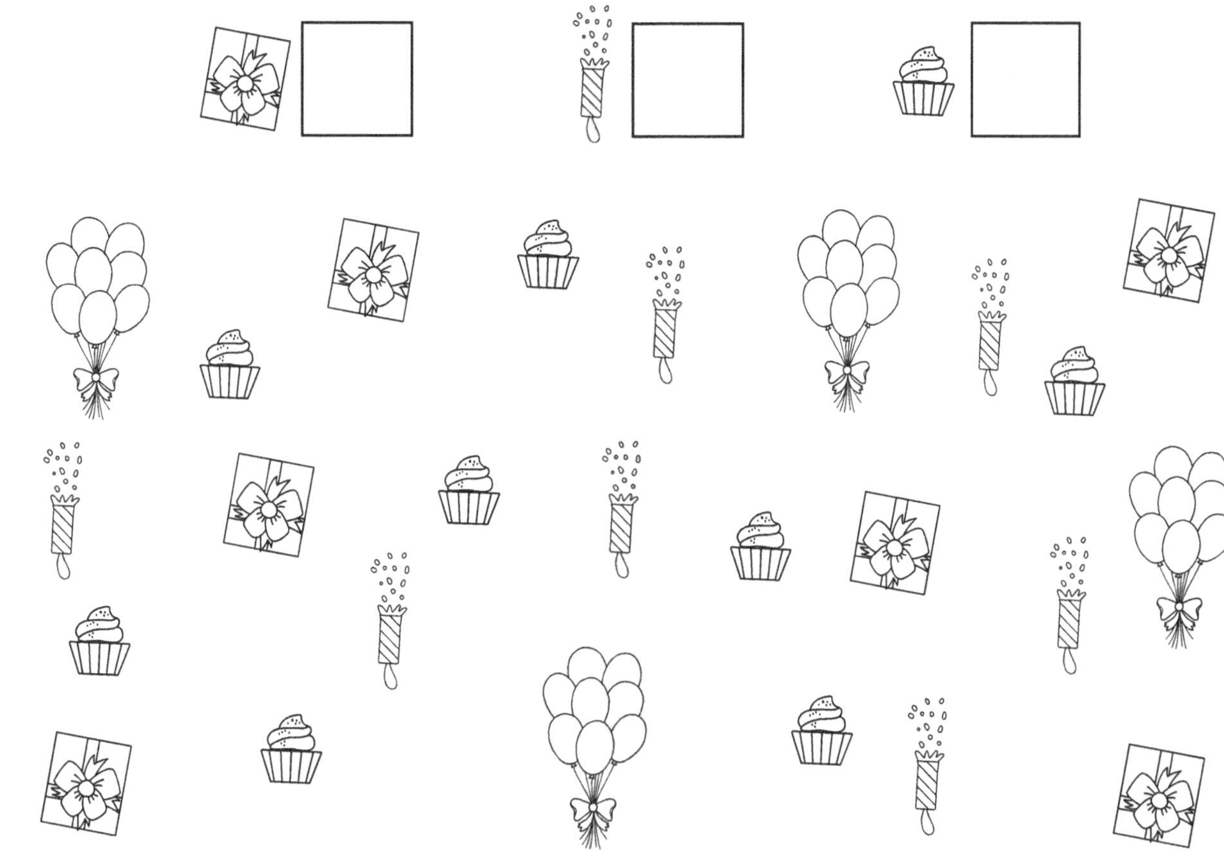

51. Connect from 1 to 11.

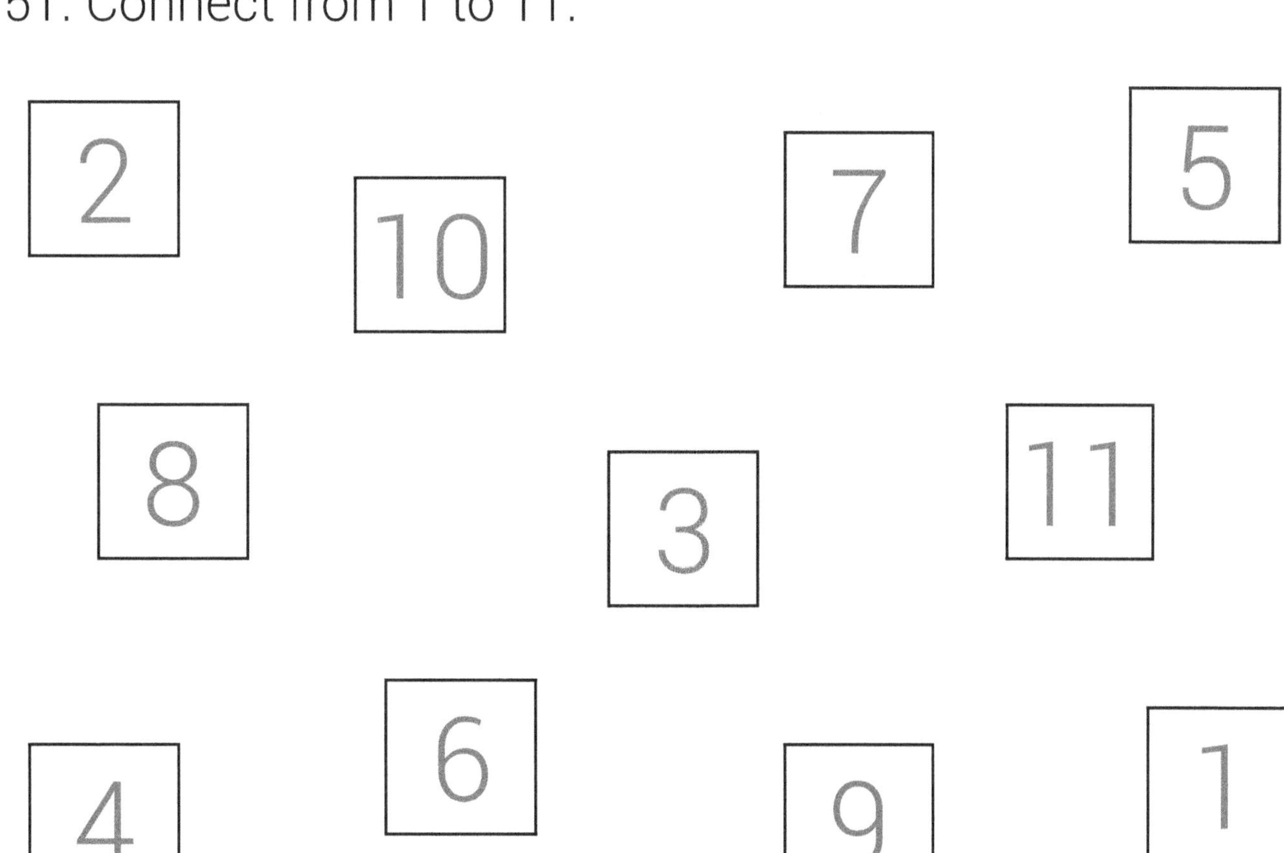

52. Write down what you see in the picture.

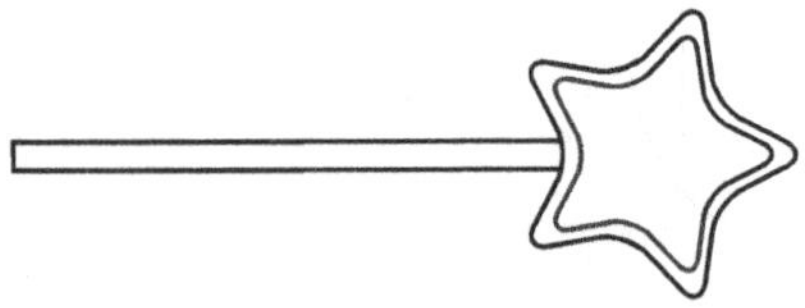

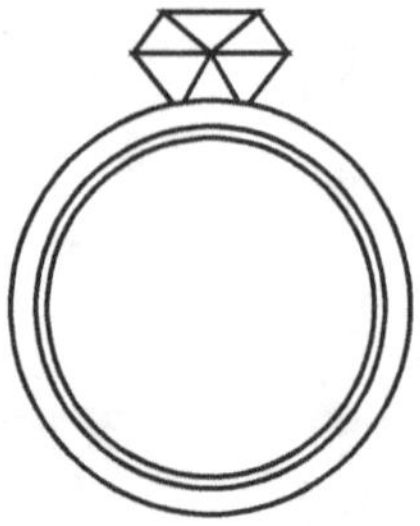

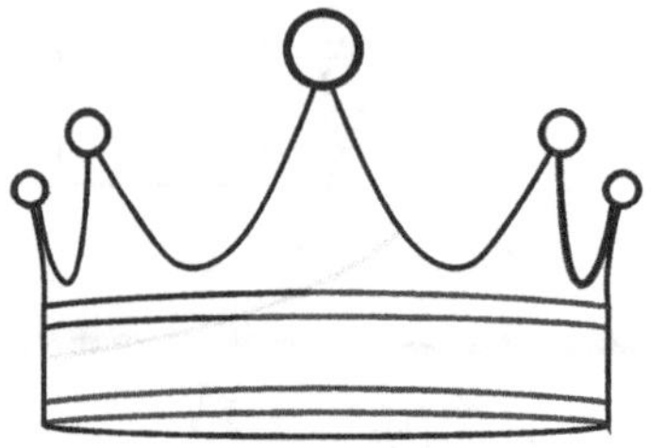

. . . .

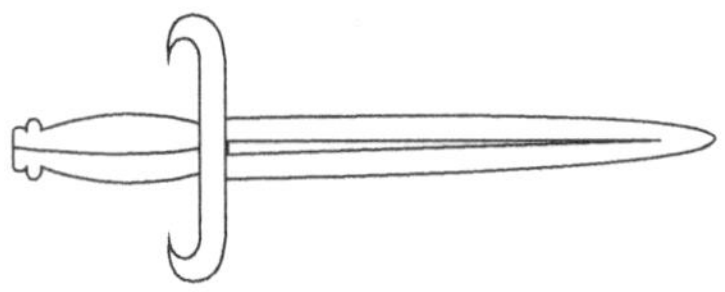

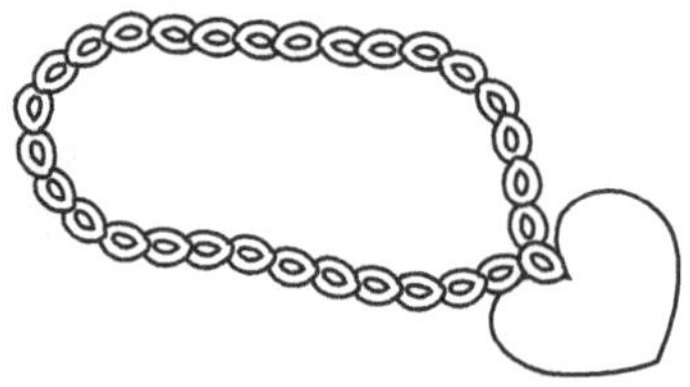

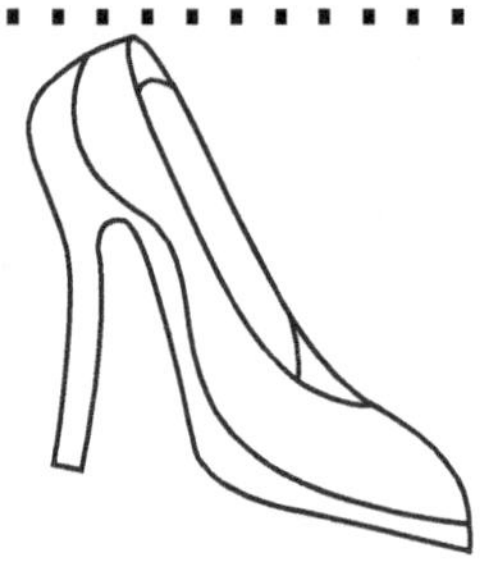

. . . .

53. Copy the picture.

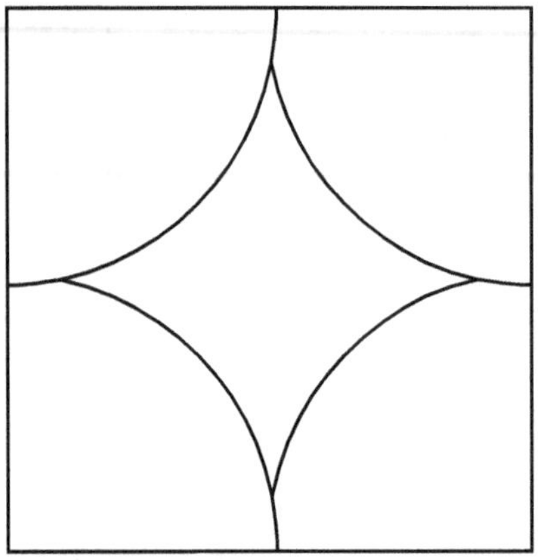

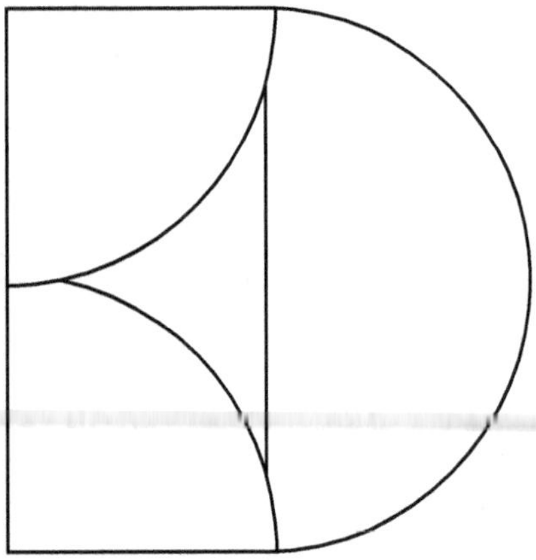

54. Read and remember, cover with your hand and write from memory.

peach pear apple	
pineapple banana coconut	

55. Matching game.

- 18:00

- 21:00

- 17:00

- 22:00

56. Counting game.

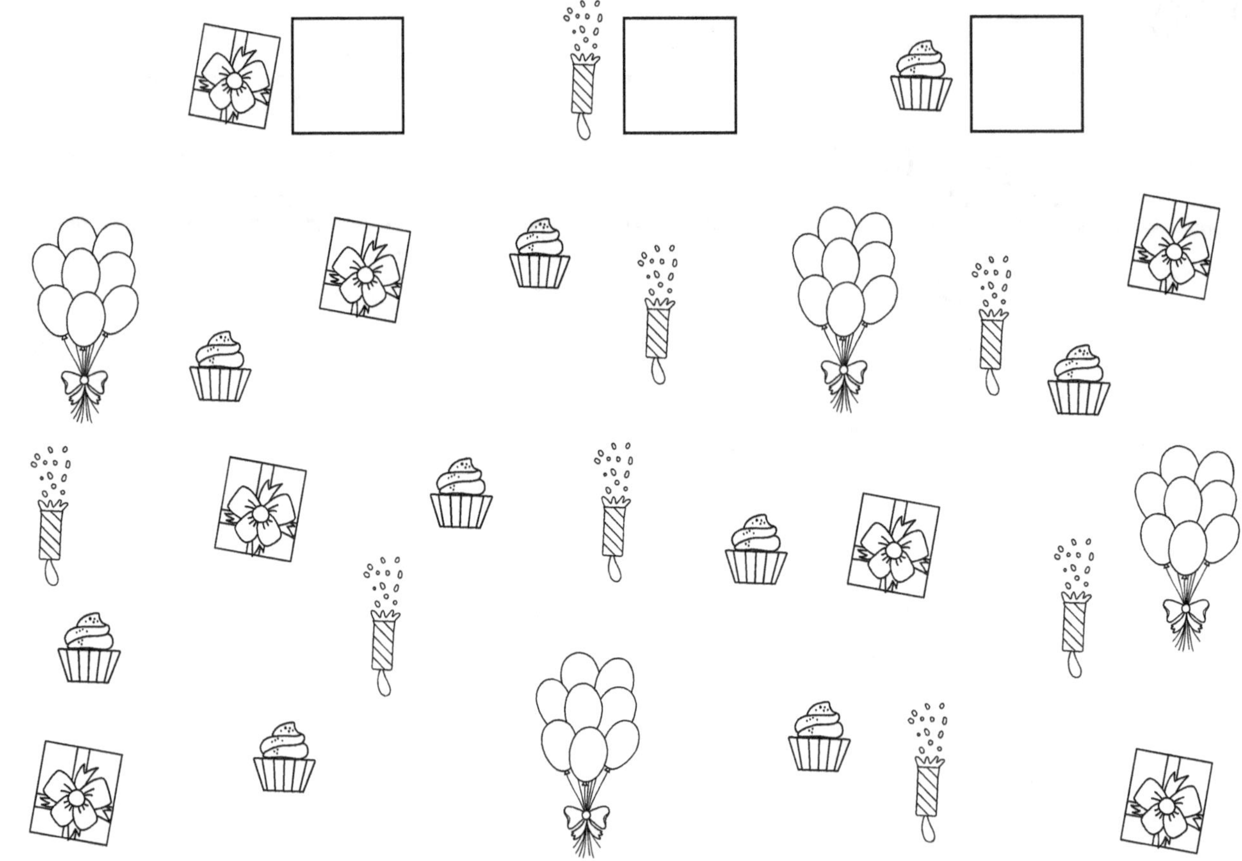

57. Write down what you see in the picture.

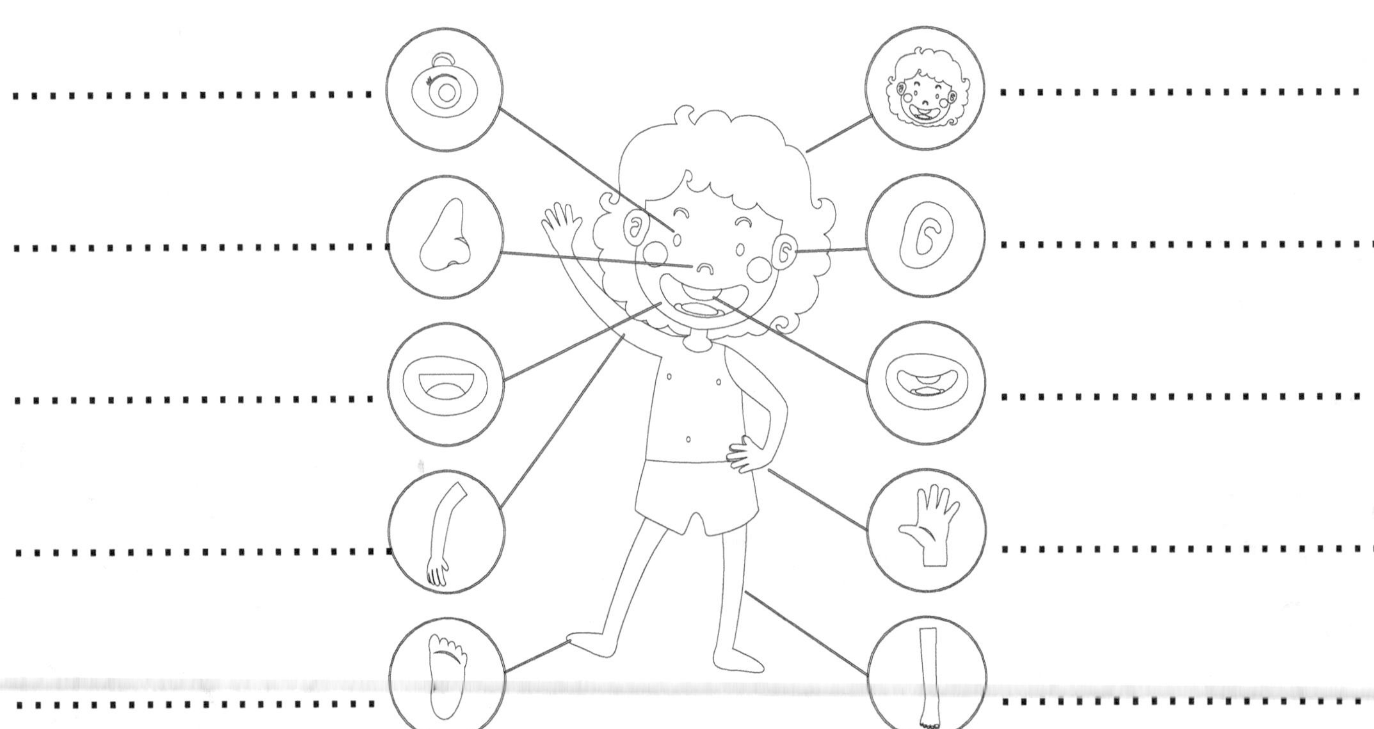

58. What is there that has no pair?

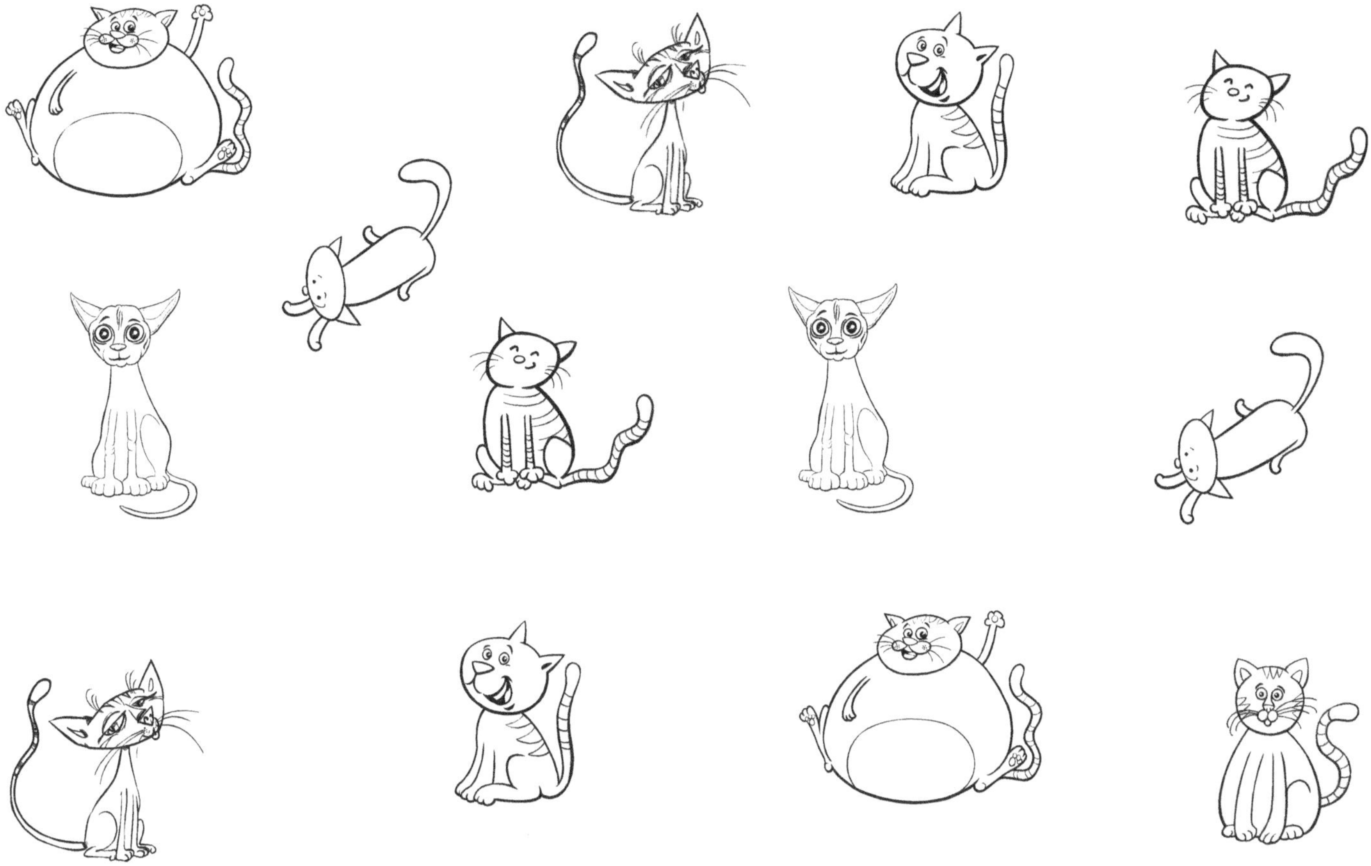

59. Copy the picture.

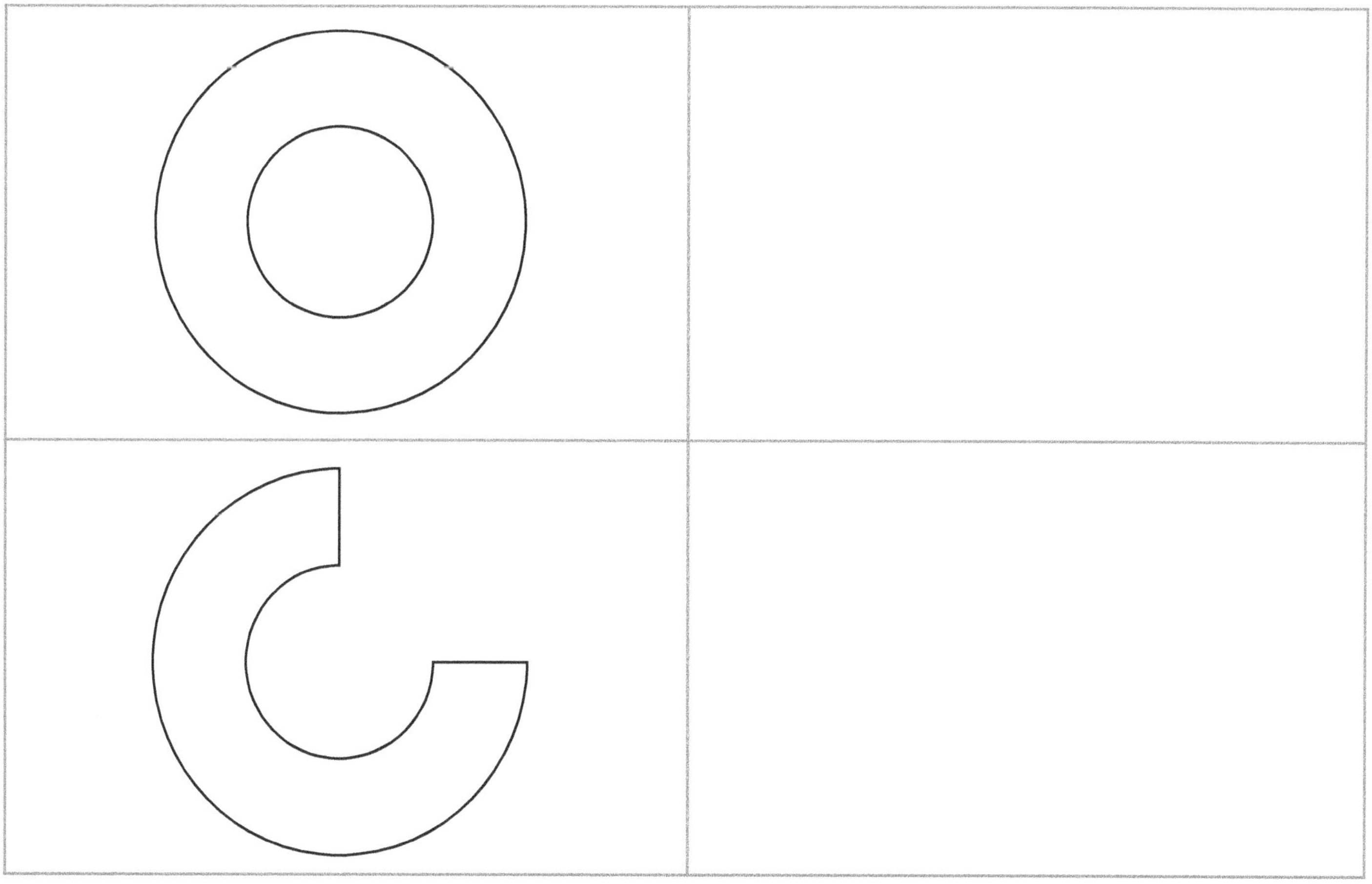

60. Read and remember, cover with your hand and write from memory.

grapes watermelon cherry	
lime lemon orange	

61. List as many words as possible from the category Wild Animals:

....

....

....

....

....

....

62. Dot to dot.

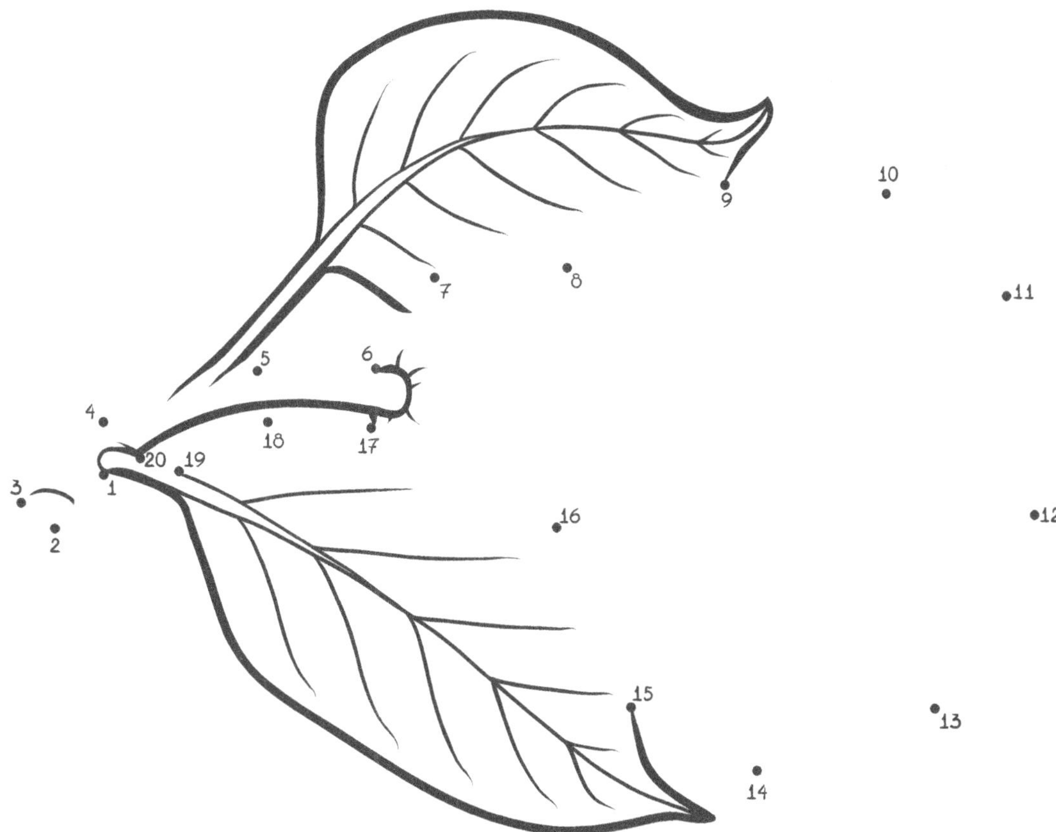

63. What season is missing there?

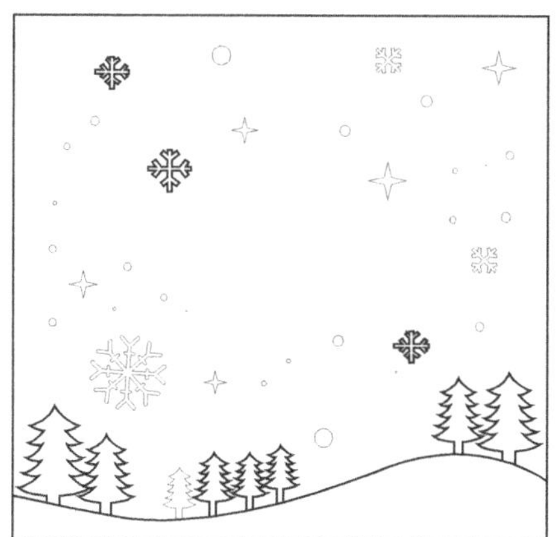

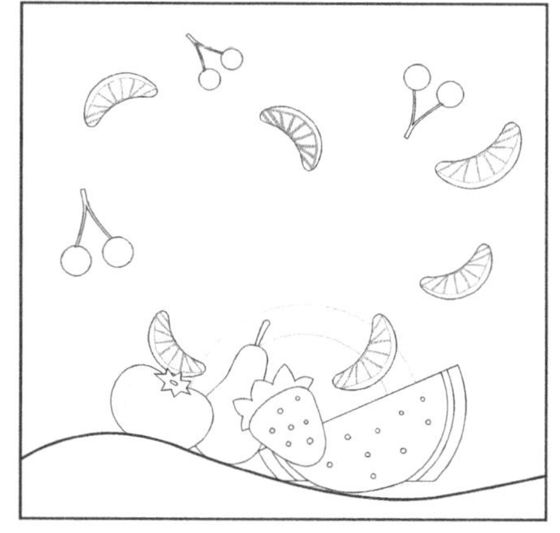

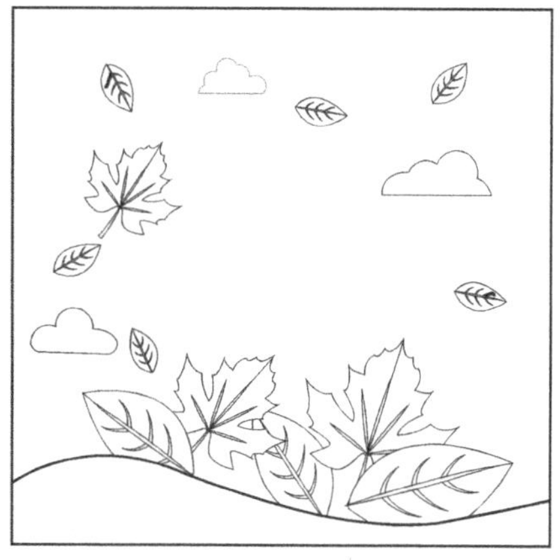

64. Copy the picture.

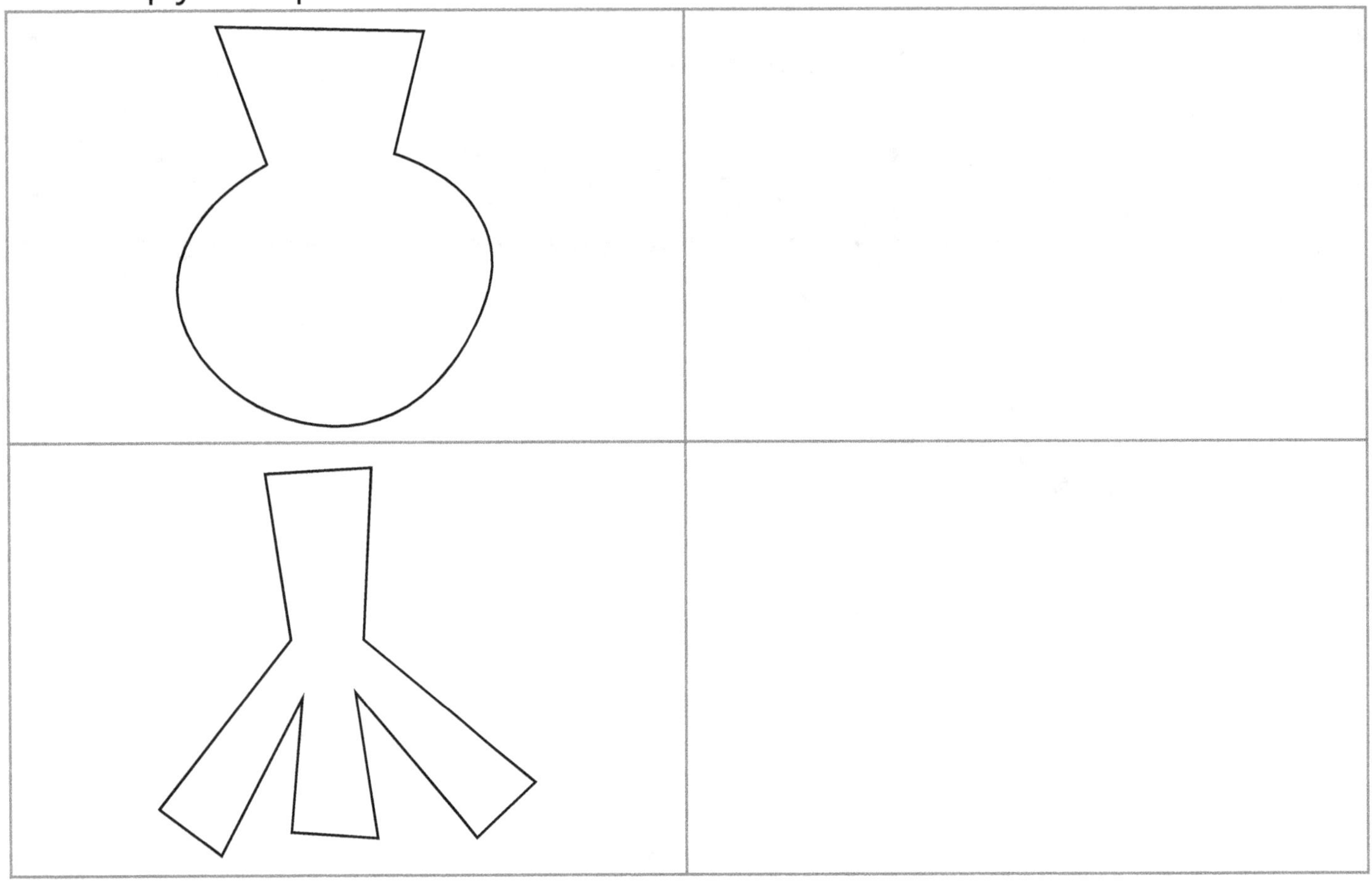

65. Read and remember, cover with your hand and write from memory.

red green blue	
yellow white pink black	

66. Counting game.

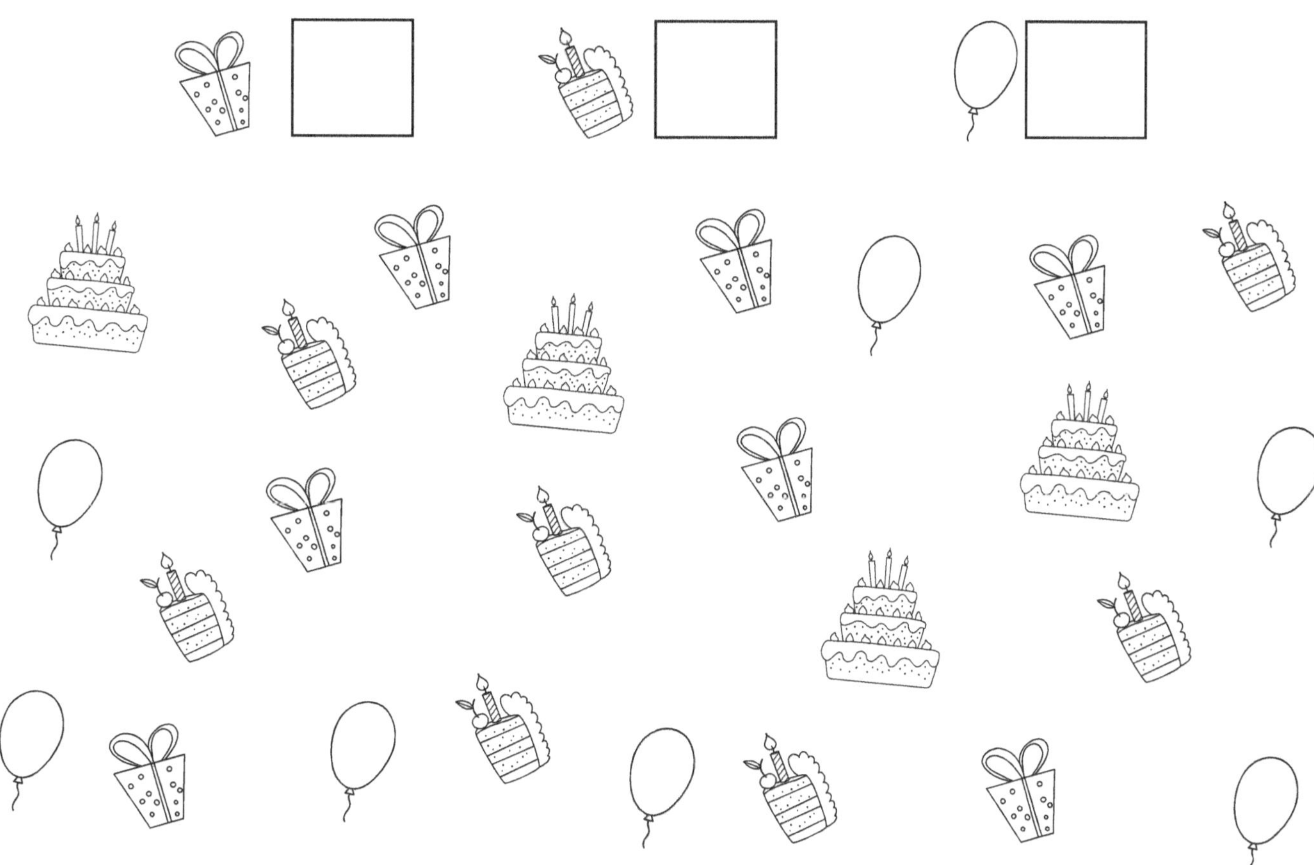 : $2 =$

: $3 =$

: $2 =$

: $4 =$

67. How many?

68. Write the number to sequence the story.

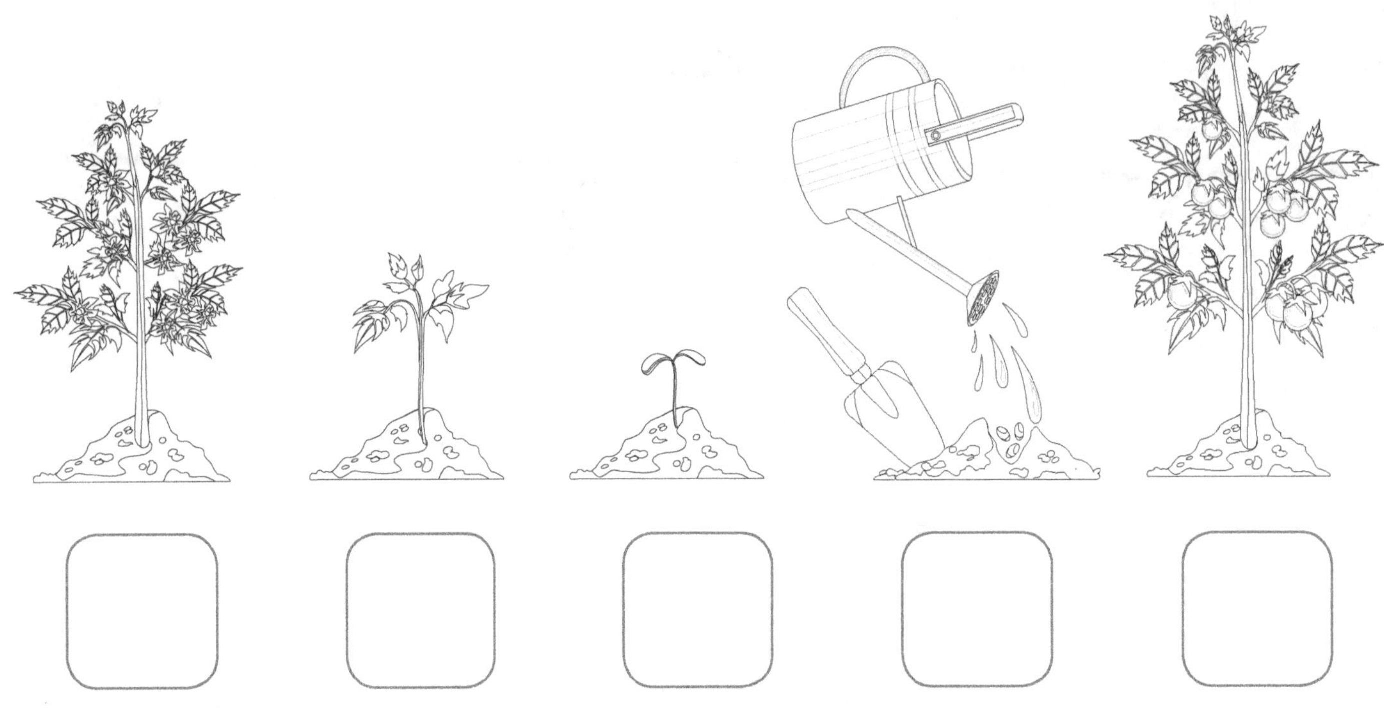

69. Find 5 differences.

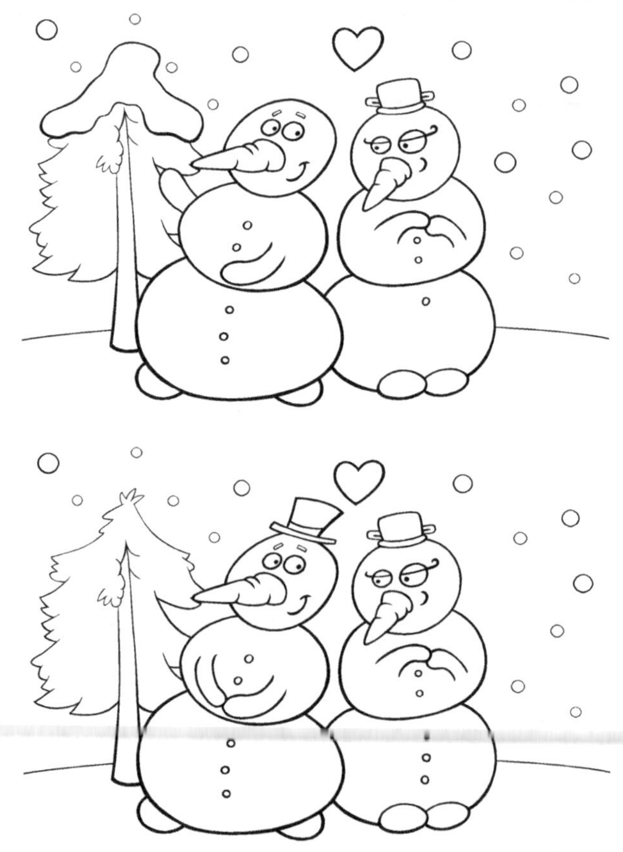

70. Match pairs.

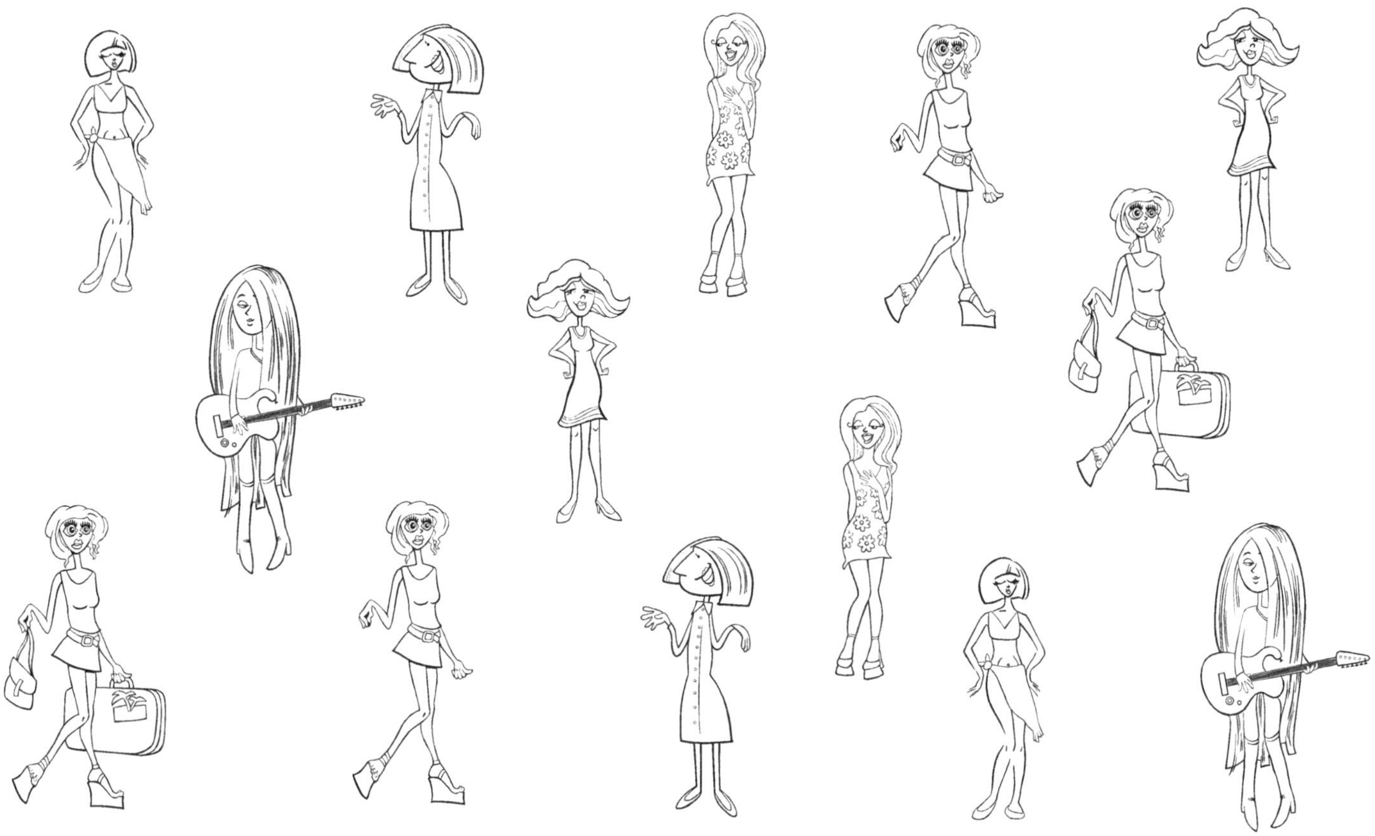

71. What does not fit?

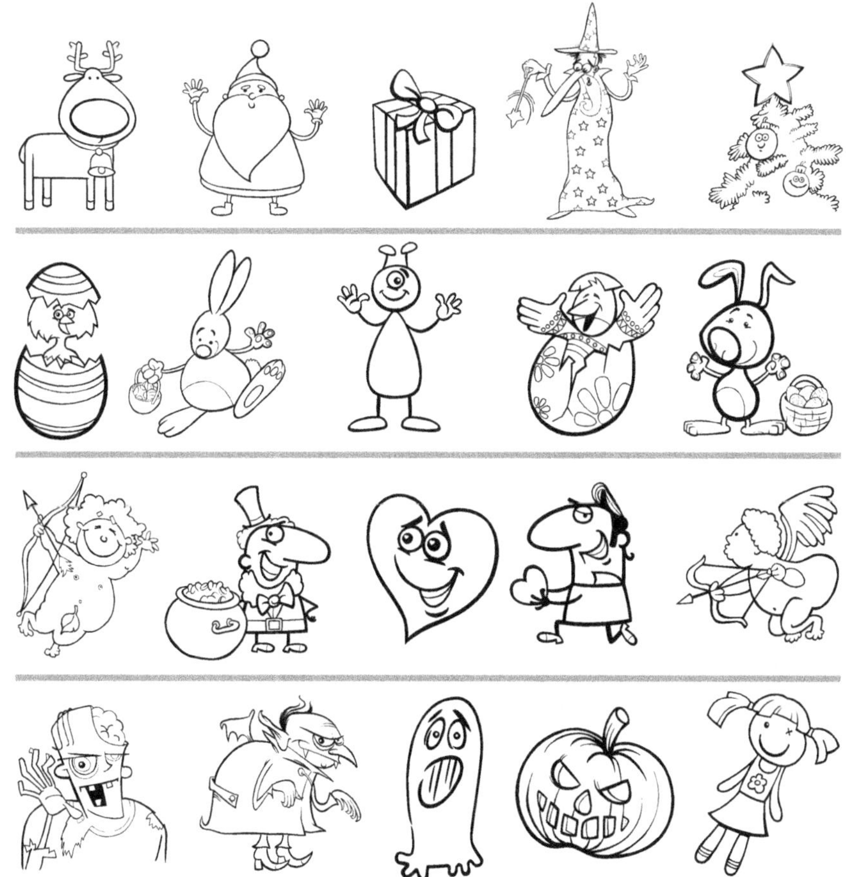

72. More or less?

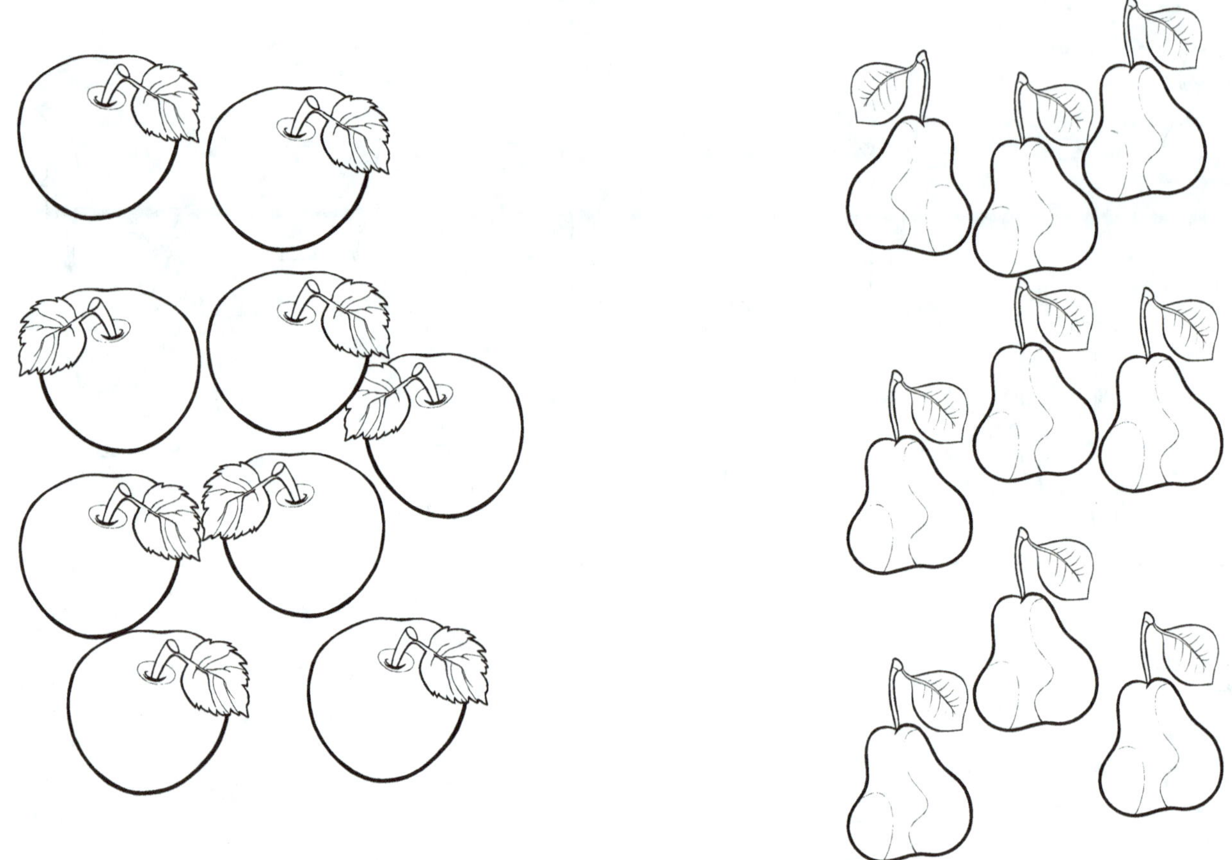

73. Write down what you see in the picture.

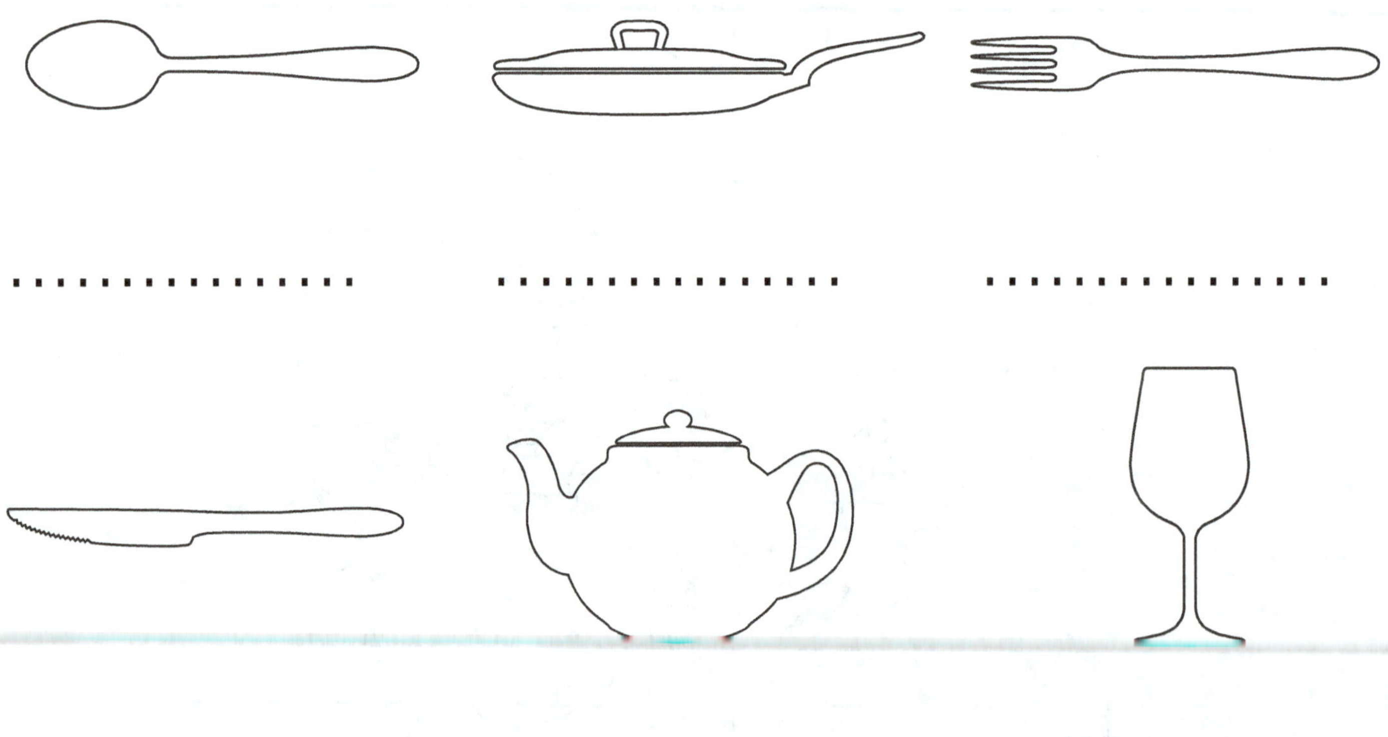

. . . .

. . . .

74. Copy the picture.

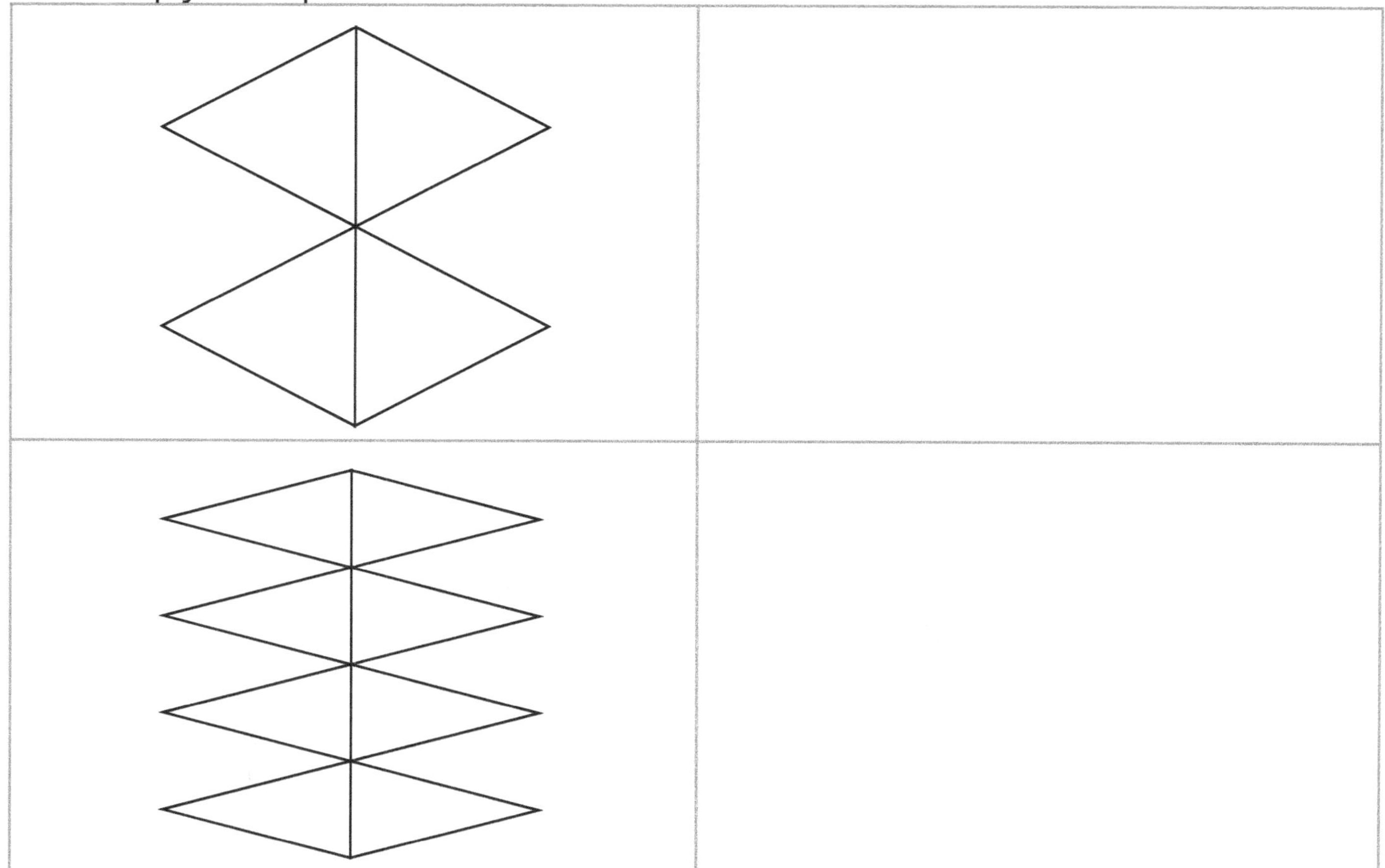

75. Counting game.

$6 + 5 =$

$5 - 3 =$

$5 \times 2 =$

$8 : 2 =$

76. Find the correct shadow.

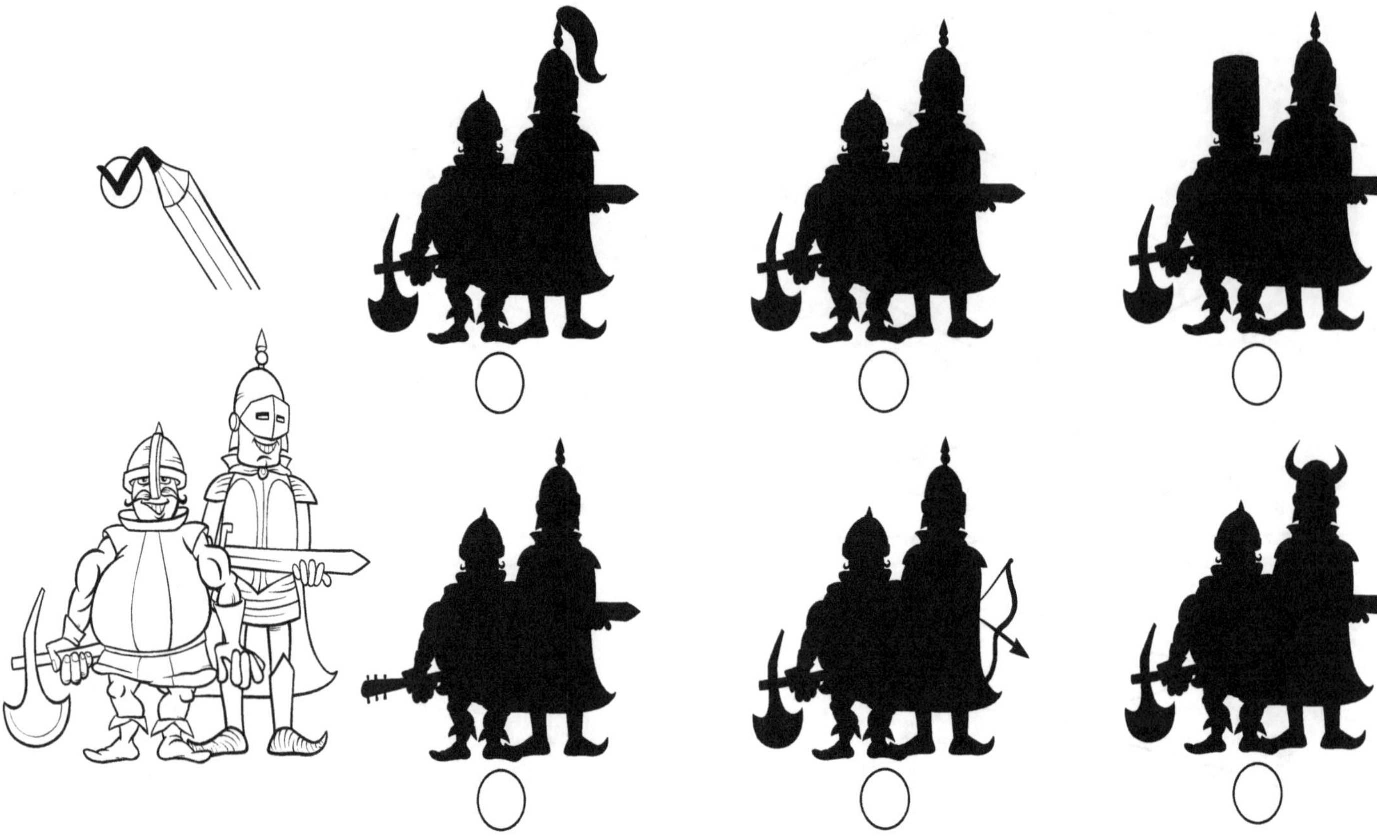

77. More or less?

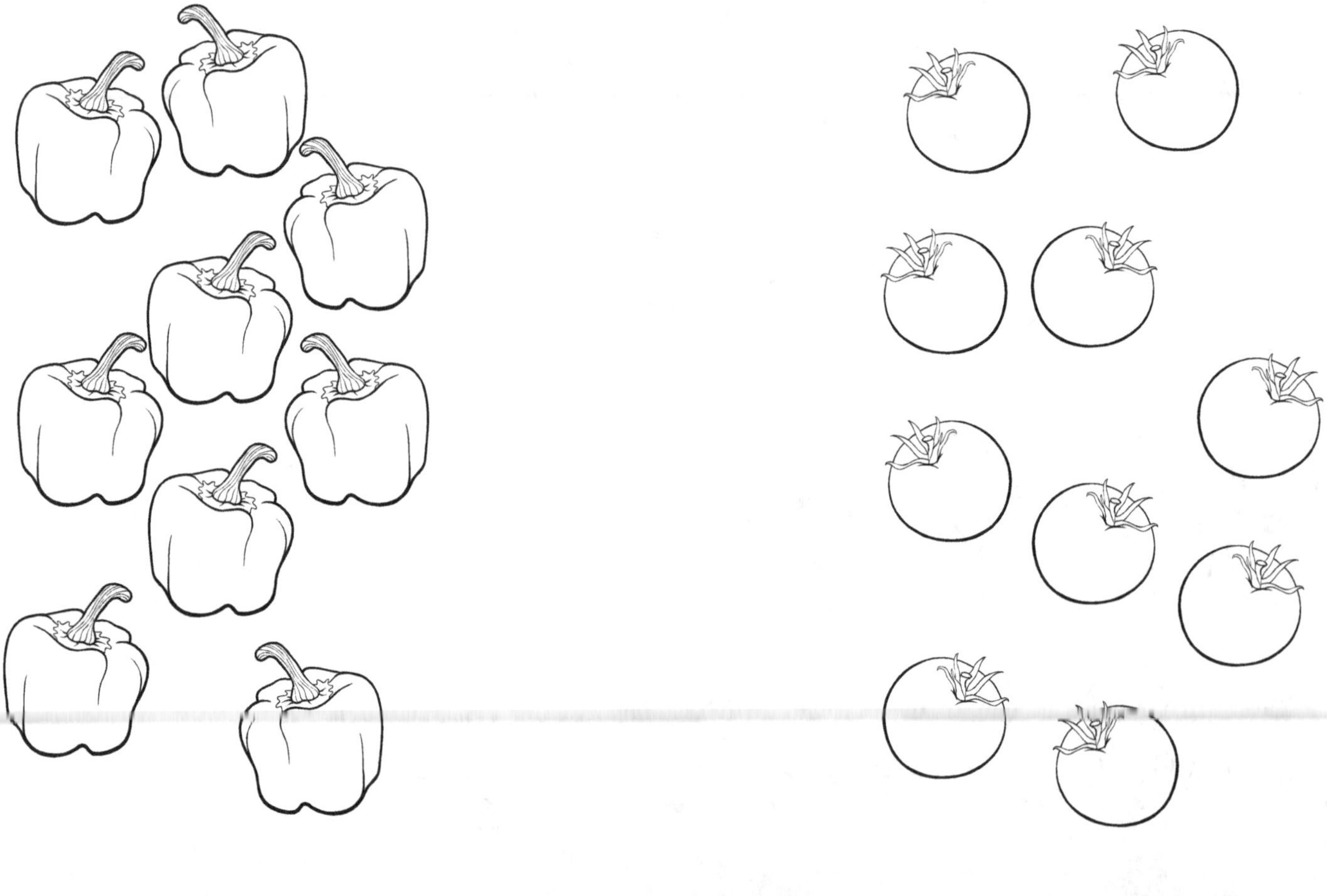

78. Dot to dot.

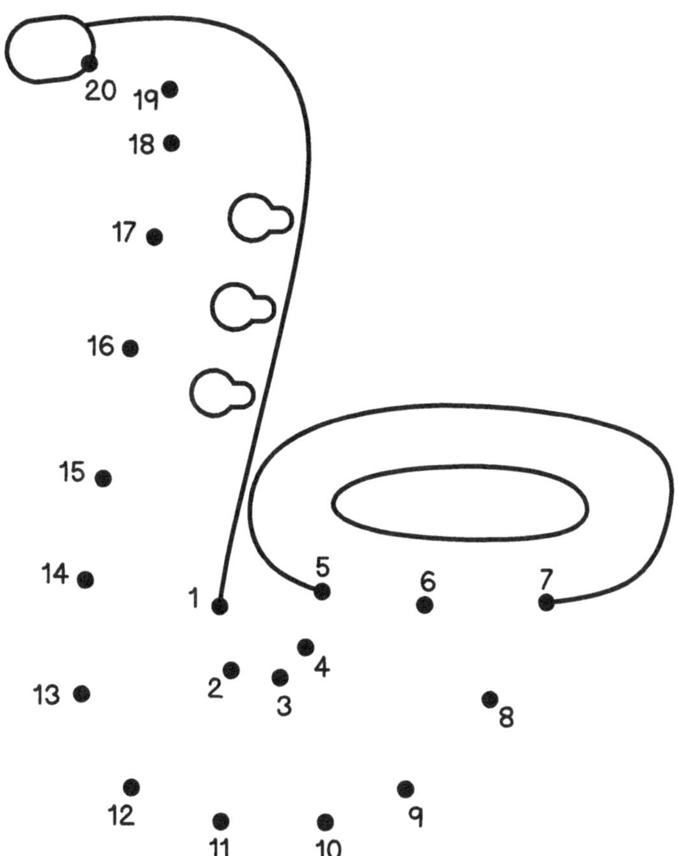

79. Word search puzzle.

X	X	R	M	M	H	N	F
A	Z	I	R	C	O	R	N
G	X	C	O	O	K	I	E
V	X	E	F	L	O	U	R
J	P	A	S	T	A	Y	G
F	R	O	B	R	E	A	D
B	U	T	T	E	R	B	C
T	O	A	S	T	B	O	E

COOKIE
TOAST
CORN
RICE
BREAD
PASTA
FLOUR
BUTTER

80. What is there that has no pair?

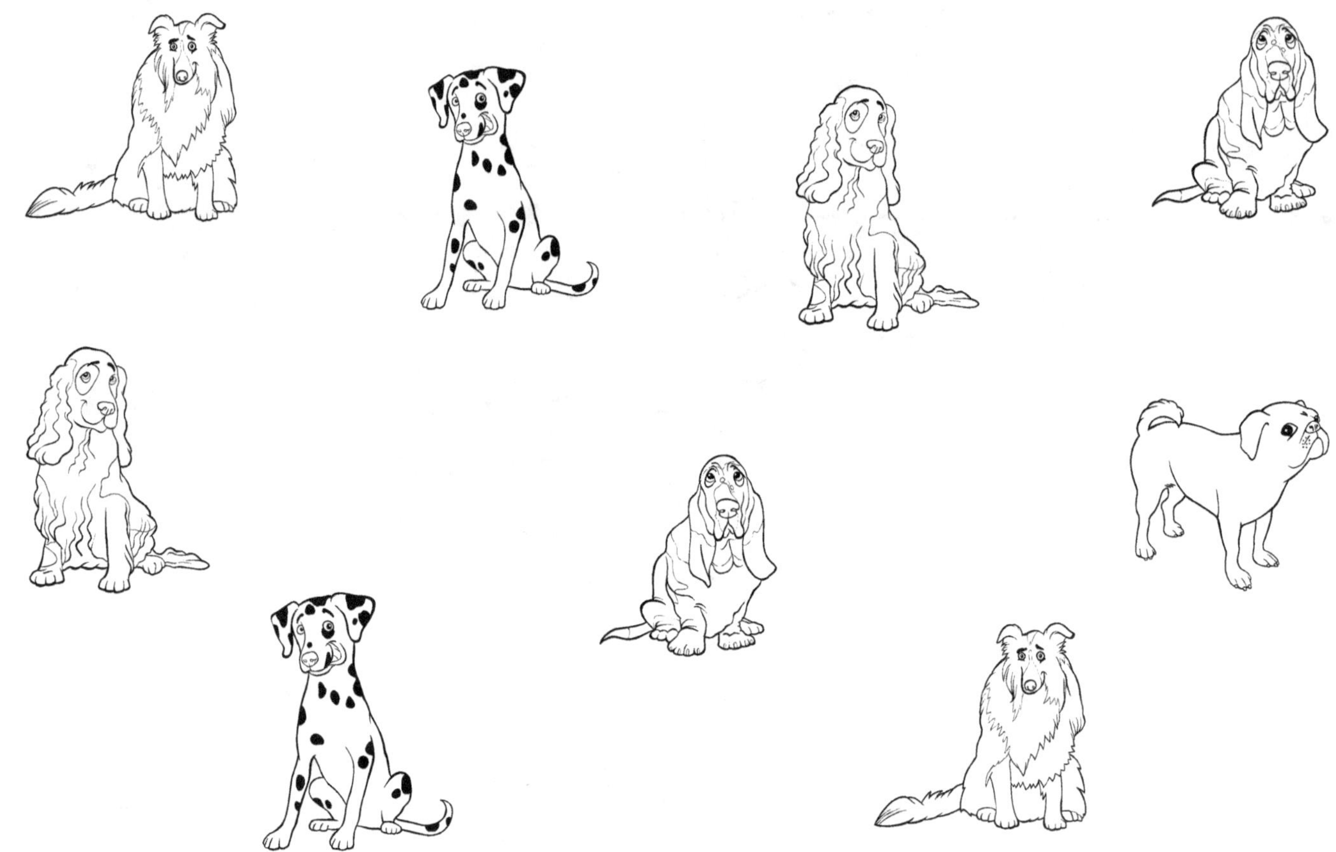

INTERMEDIATE LEVEL

1. Dot to dot.

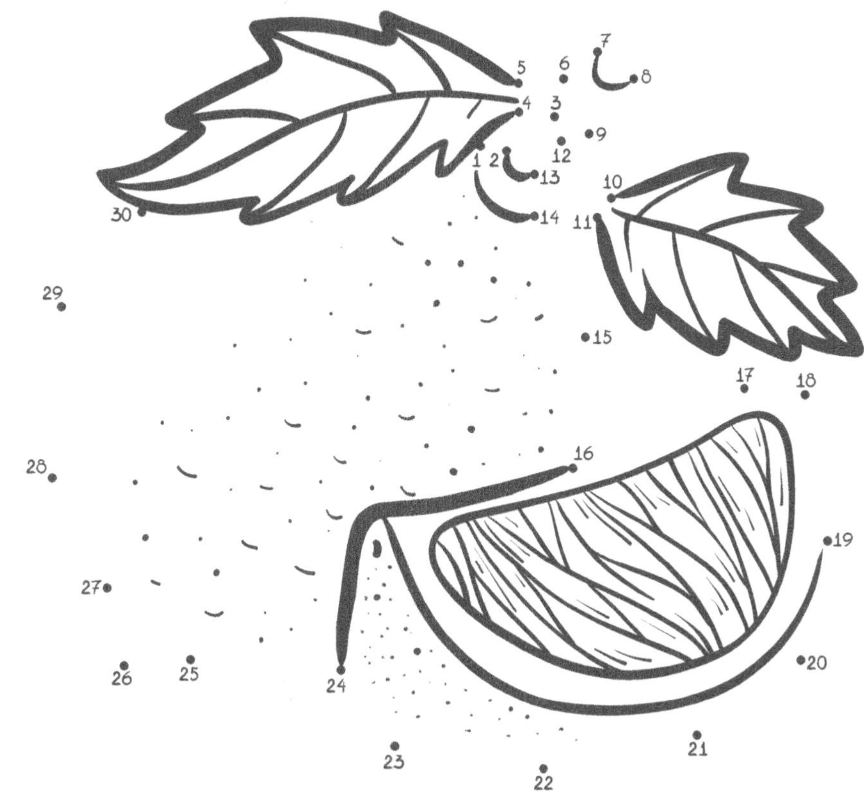

2. Counting game.

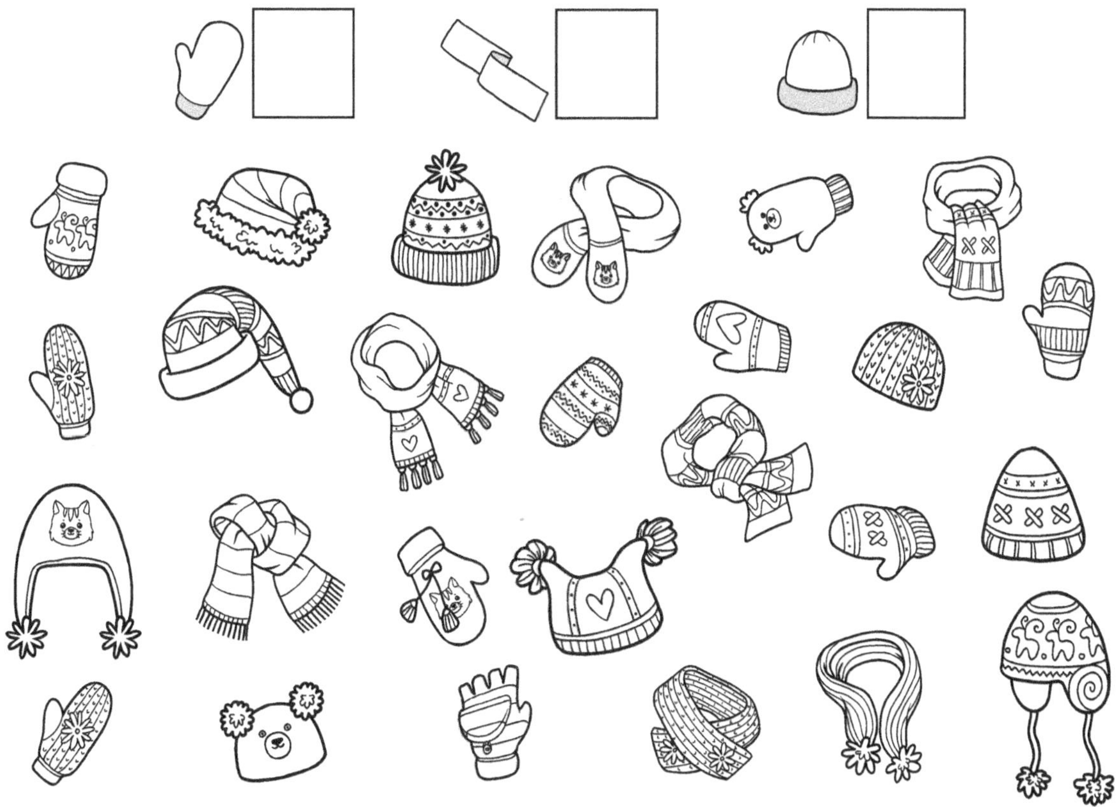

3. Find 6 differences.

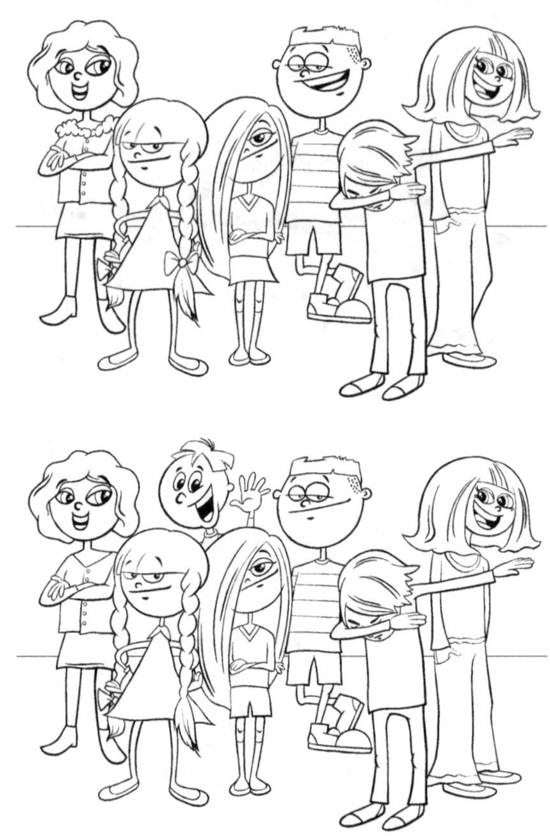

4. What are the synonyms for the words:

Holiday	Food
. . . .	. . . .
. . . .	. . . .
. . . .	. . . .
. . . .	. . . .
. . . .	. . . .

5. Name as many yellow fruits and vegetables as you can.

....

....

....

....

....

6. Word search puzzle.

A	F	I	R	E	P	L	A	C	E	I
X	T	C	U	X	W	A	C	N	C	M
K	Q	G	X	Y	H	B	O	I	I	B
P	T	A	H	R	O	H	U	A	F	O
H	V	L	I	A	V	I	G	Q	R	U
S	S	E	Y	D	E	C	H	W	O	U
N	S	S	R	I	R	I	P	S	S	R
O	N	L	T	A	C	C	N	K	T	P
W	X	E	M	T	O	L	O	A	Y	I
M	B	D	F	O	A	E	Z	T	G	C
A	X	G	U	R	T	S	Y	E	F	E
N	I	E	F	R	I	R	Q	S	Z	N

COUGH
FIREPLACE
FROSTY
ICE
SKATES
ICICLE
OVERCOAT
RADIATOR
SLEDGE
SNOWMAN
GALE

7. What is there that has no pair?

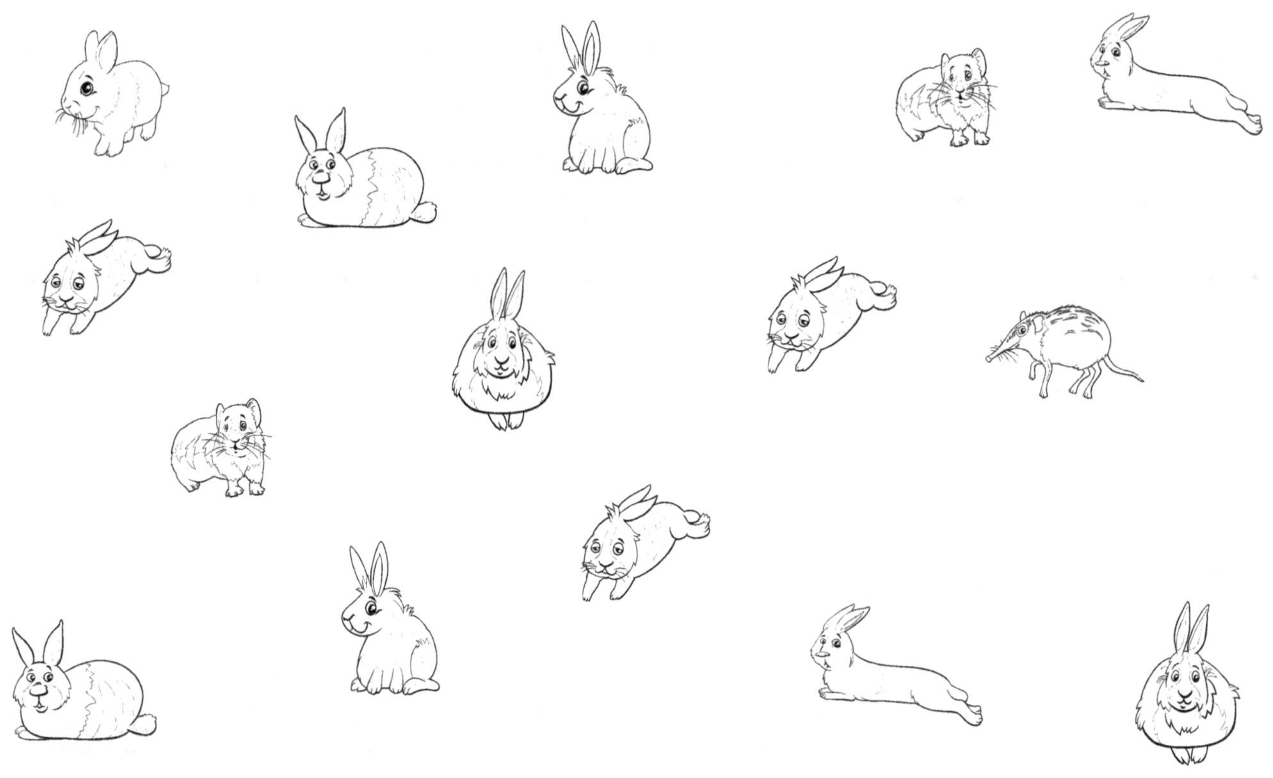

8. What would be useful for a gardener?

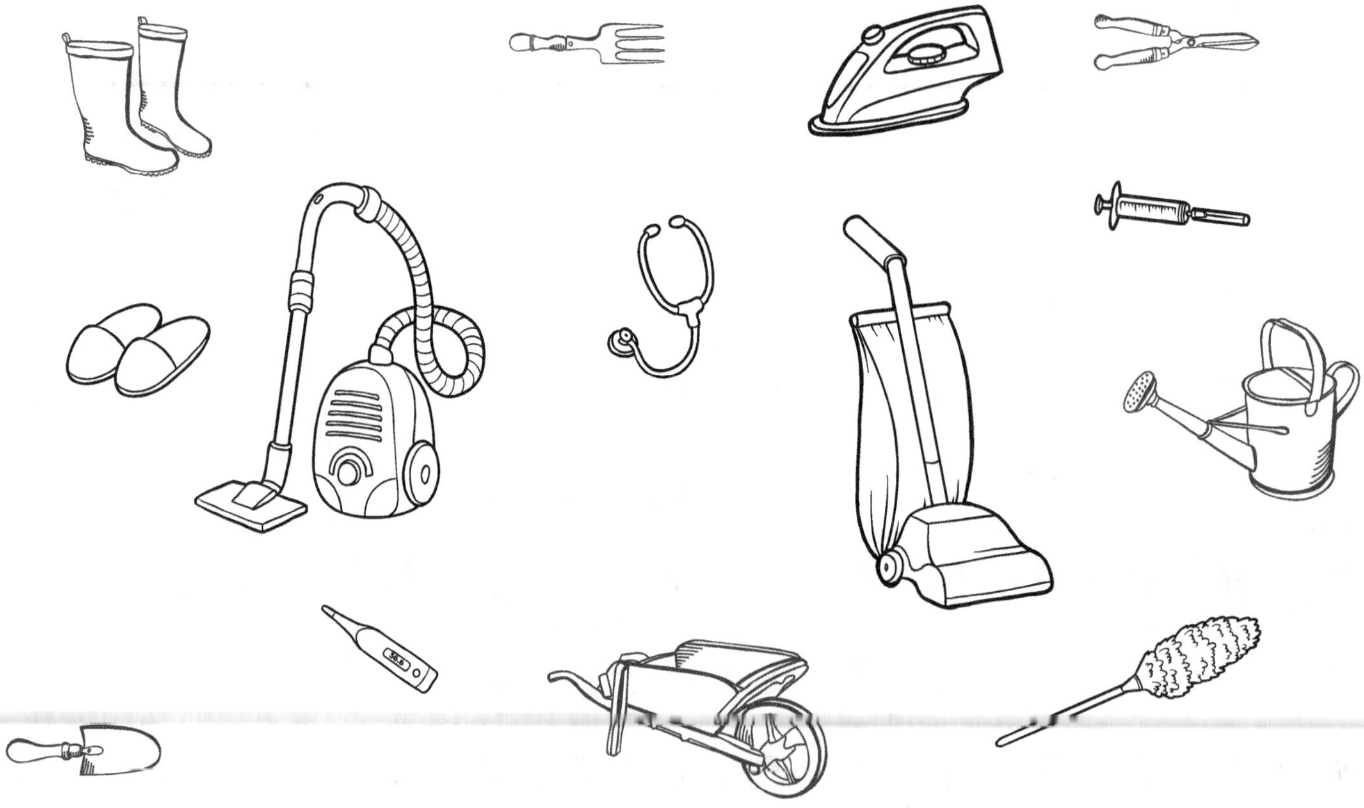

9. List as many words as possible from the category Mushrooms:

....

....

....

....

....

....

10. Write down all the words that you know describing the word -Hair:

....

....

....

....

....

11. More or less?

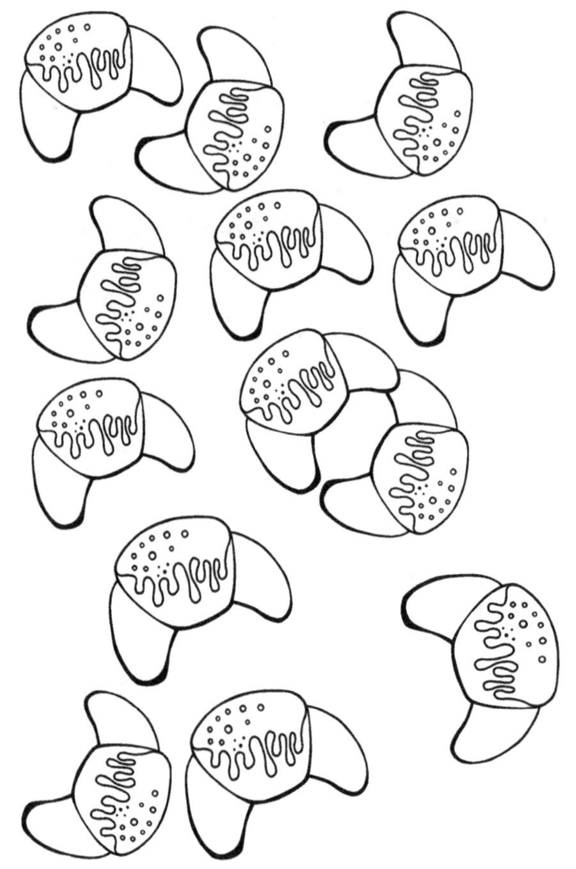 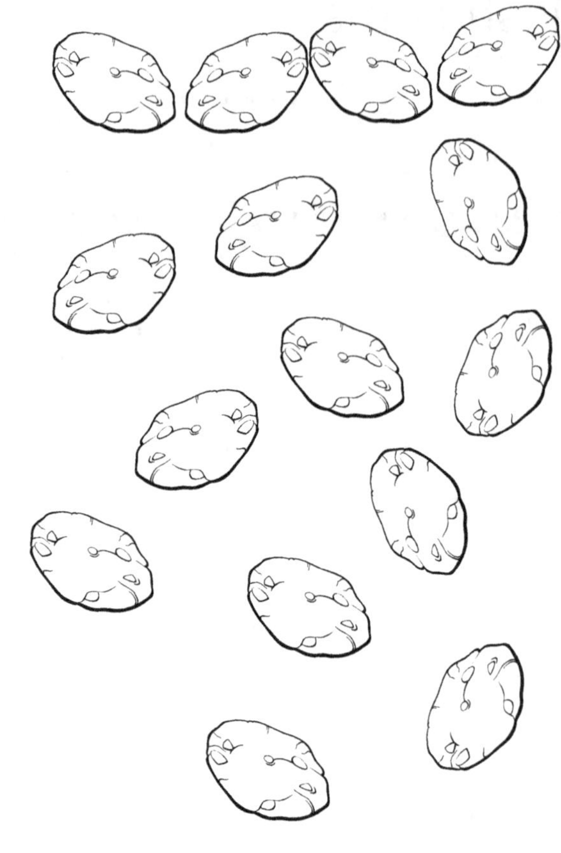

12. Counting game.

$4+6=...$ $\qquad$ $23+6=...$

$5+6=...$ $\qquad$ $35+5=...$

$8+9=...$ $\qquad$ $18+3=...$

$7+9=...$ $\qquad$ $27+4=...$

$11+6=...$ $\qquad$ $11+11=...$

$12+7=...$ $\qquad$ $12+9=...$

$11+12=...$ $\qquad$ $11+12=...$

13. Dot to dot.

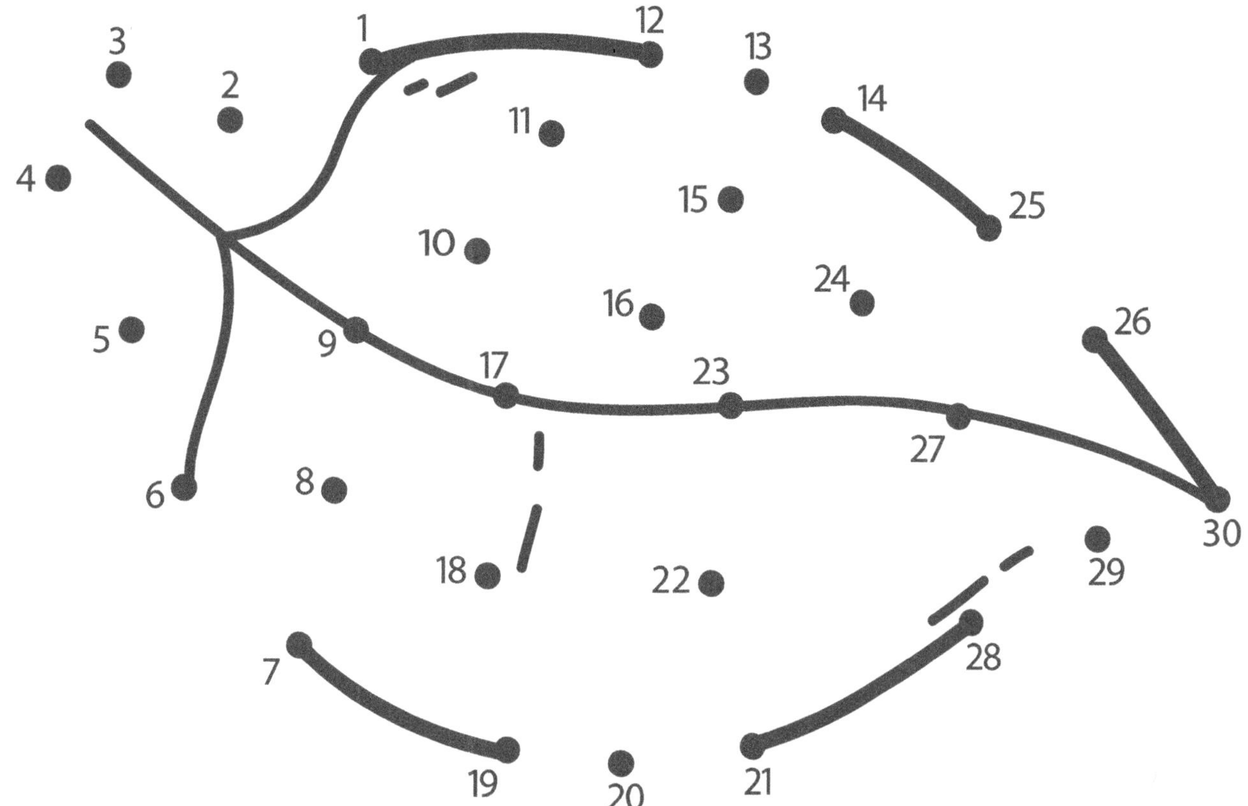

14. Read and remember, cover with your hand and write from memory.

12 14 16 18	
26 28 32 34	

15. Name the shoes and write down what seasons of the year we wear them.

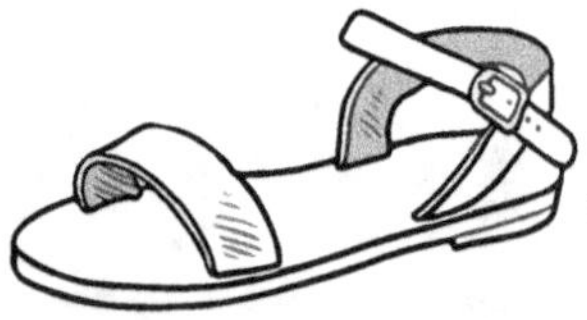

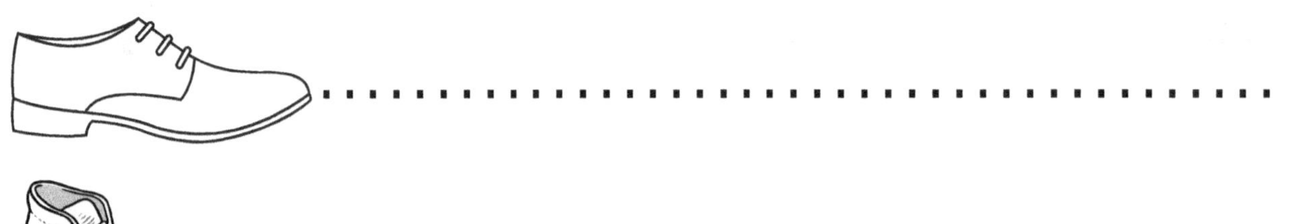

....

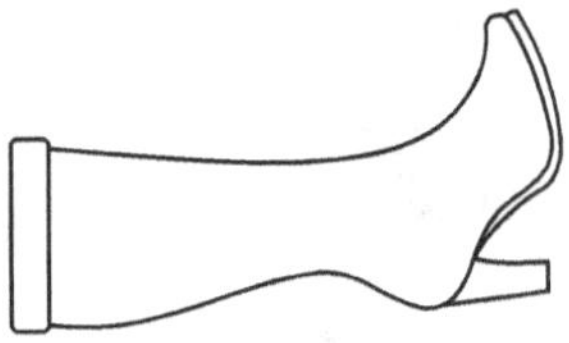

....

....

....

16. Copy the picture.

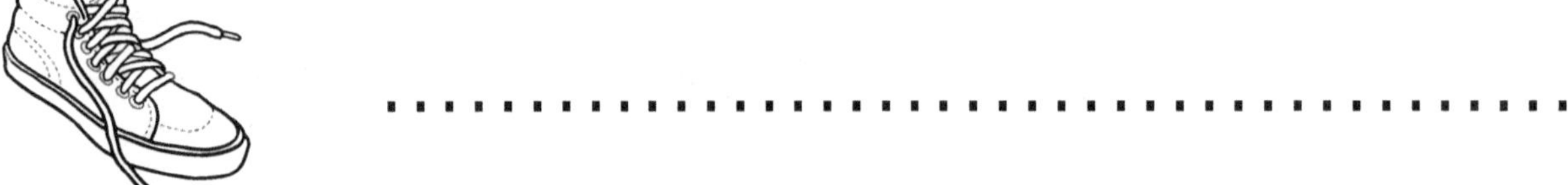

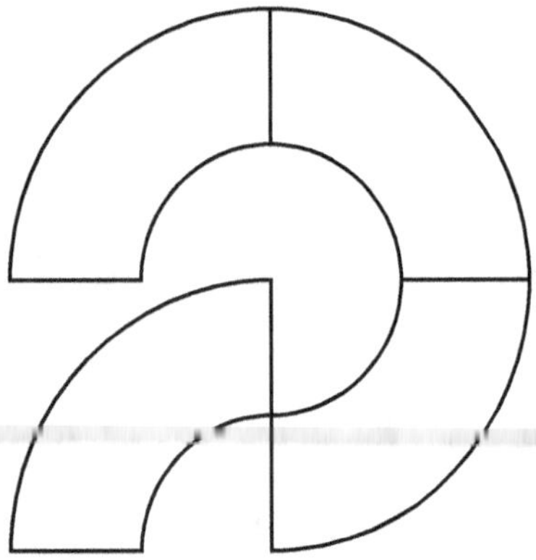

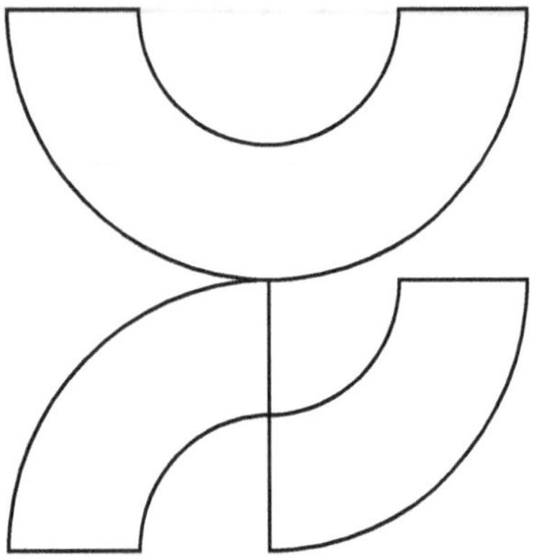

17. Write down what you see in the picture.

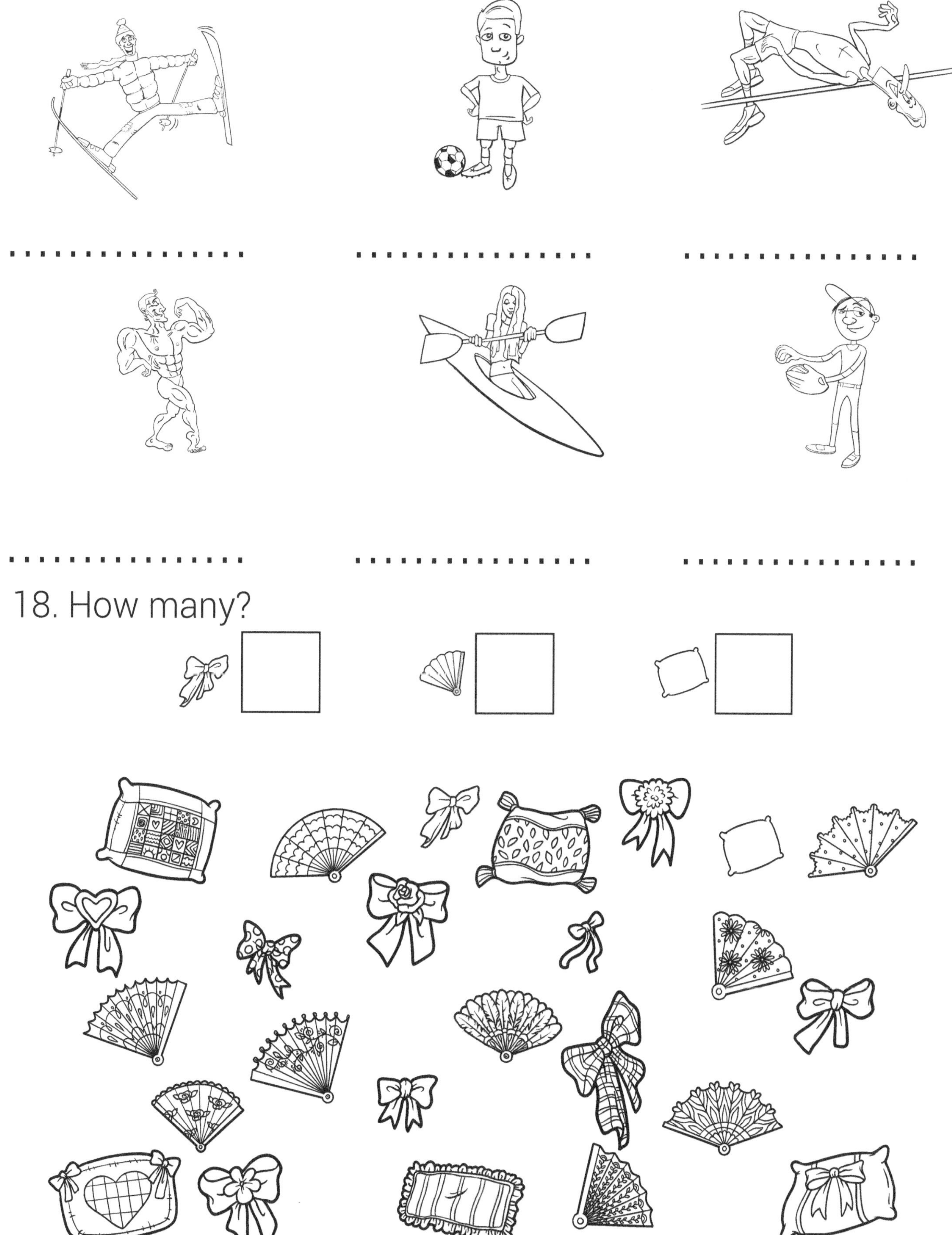

. . . .

. . . .

18. How many?

19. More or less?

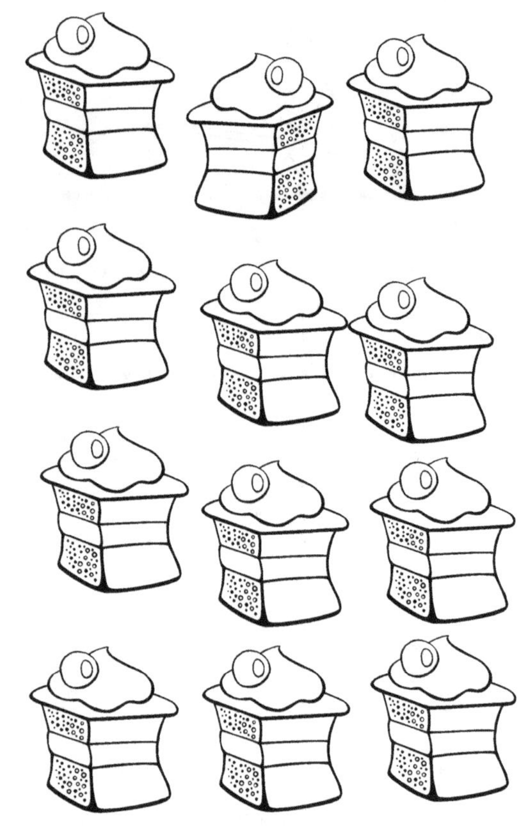
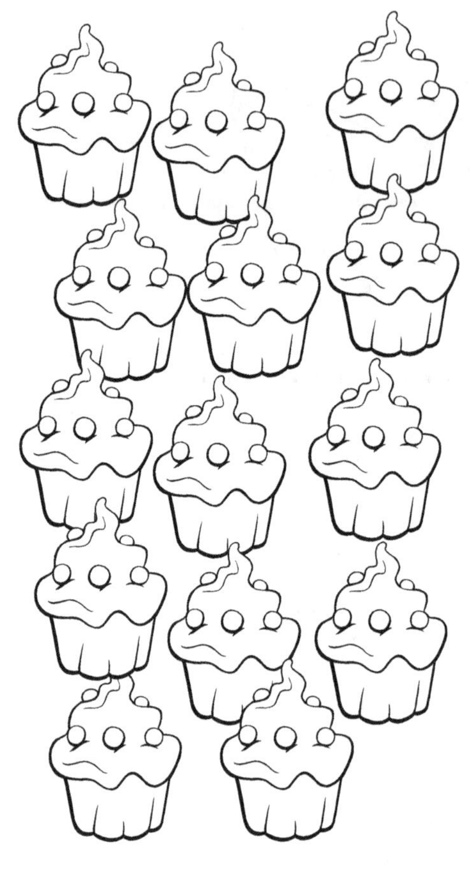

20. Complete the words.

APPL_

TAB_ _

HOUS_

FLOW_ _

BUTTERF_ _

CARRO _

POTA_ _

SHOPPI_ _

BUTT_ _

CHEE_ _

21. Counting game.

8-6=...	18-9=...
7-5=...	17-8=...
8-4=...	18-8=...
9-7=	9-7=
11-6=	81-6=
12-7=	12-7=
11-5=	21-5=

22. List as many words as possible from the category Birds:

....

....

....

....

....

23. Write down what professions you associate these items with.

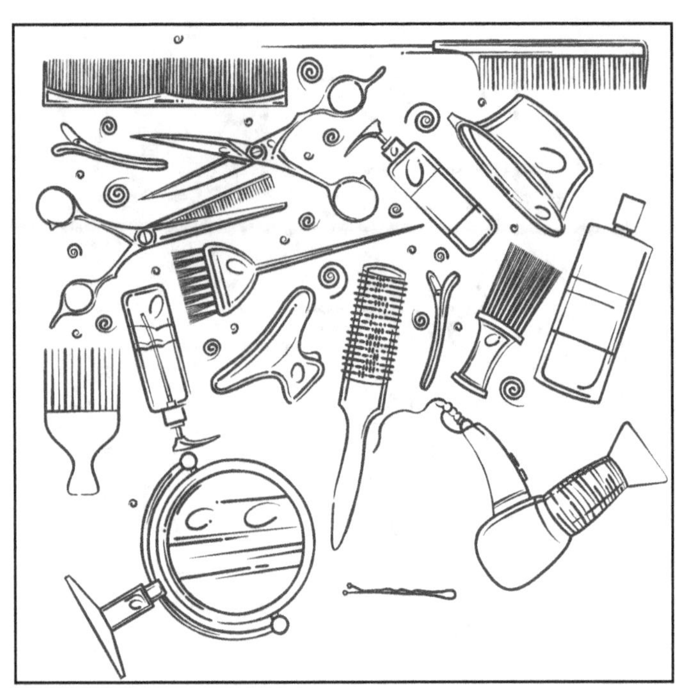 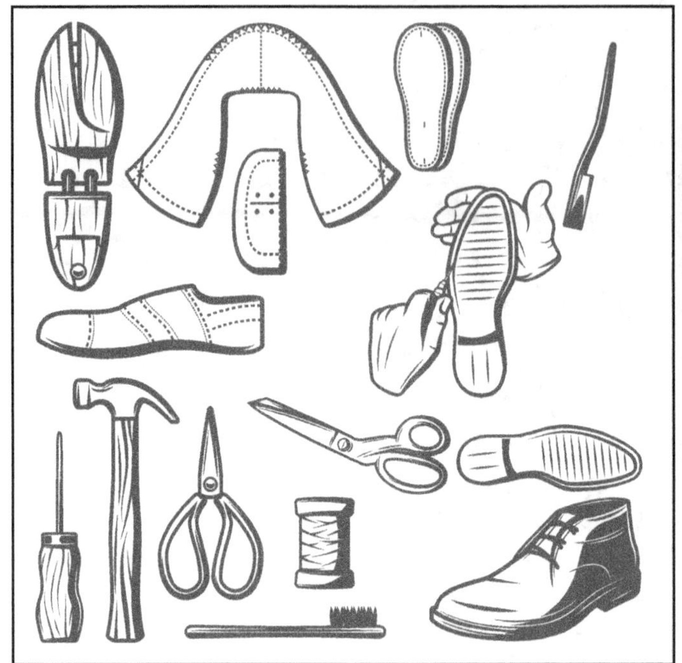

. . . .

24. Write down all the words that you know describing the word -Skirt:

. . . .

. . . .

. . . .

. . . .

. . . .

. . . .

25. Find 7 differences.

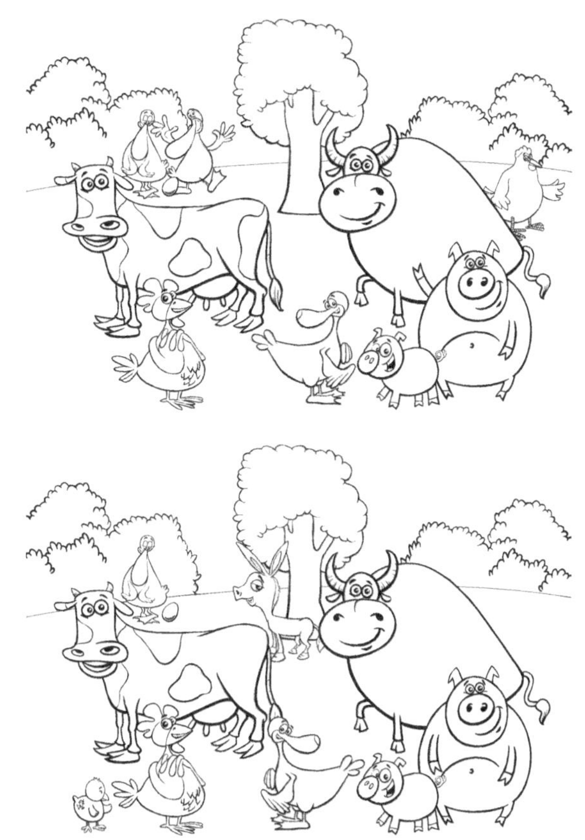

26. More or less?

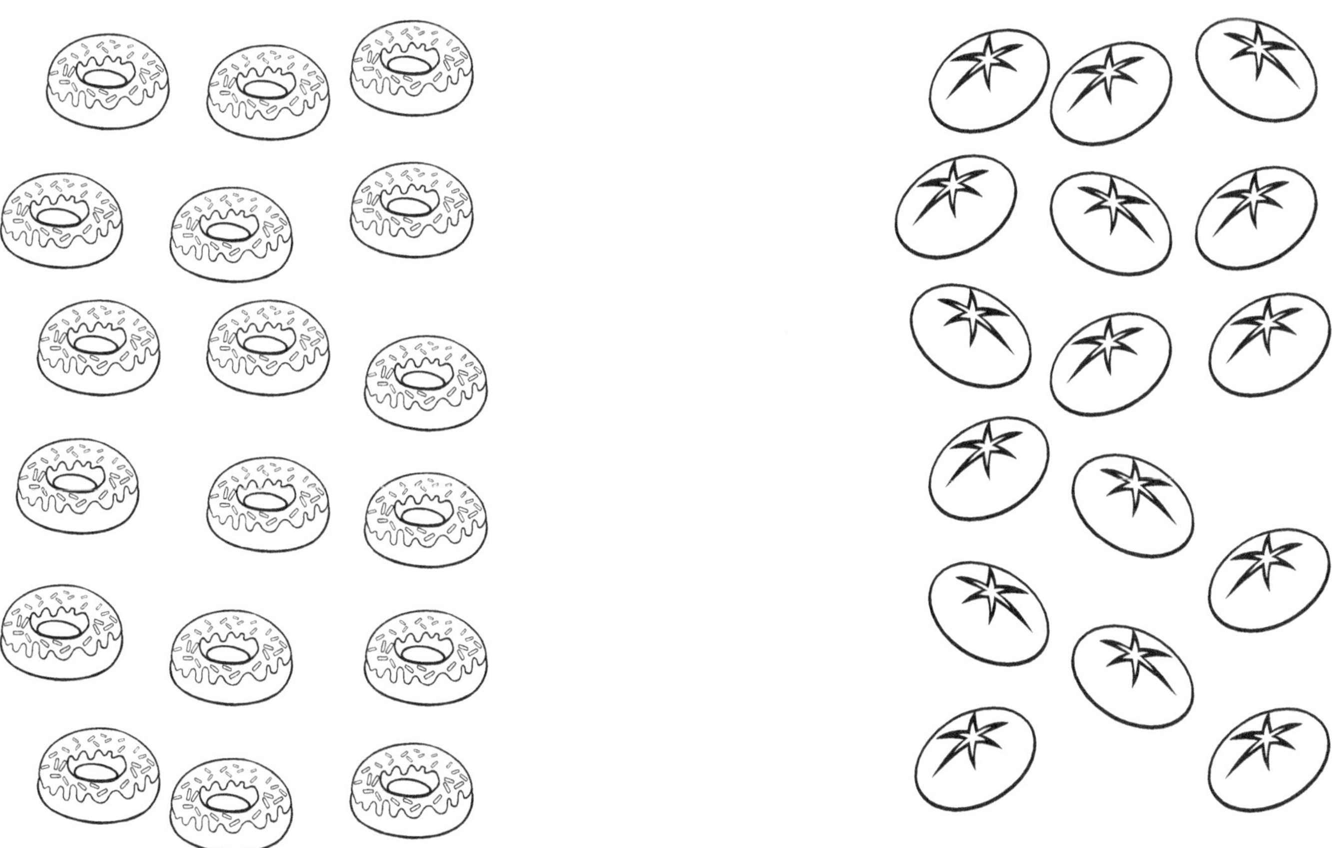

27. Word search puzzle.

F	U	Q	P	X	H	Y	N	G	O	N
D	S	S	C	P	L	U	Z	G	S	Y
G	W	H	L	T	A	F	U	O	N	K
R	A	G	E	B	D	R	I	R	O	C
A	L	J	A	Z	Y	T	P	I	W	I
S	L	M	S	Y	B	U	C	D	D	Q
S	O	C	T	R	I	L	H	A	R	R
Y	W	B	E	X	R	I	I	I	O	M
M	P	J	R	J	D	P	R	S	P	G
K	B	P	B	W	K	U	P	Y	C	Y
Y	R	L	S	E	G	G	R	M	B	W
Z	Z	H	B	U	N	N	Y	F	R	B

BUNNY
CHIRP
DAISY
EASTER
LADYBIRD
SNOWDROP
SWALLOW
TULIP
EGG
GRASS

28. Name as many green vegetables as you can.

....

....

....

....

....

29. What are the synonyms for the words:

Old	Young

30. How many?

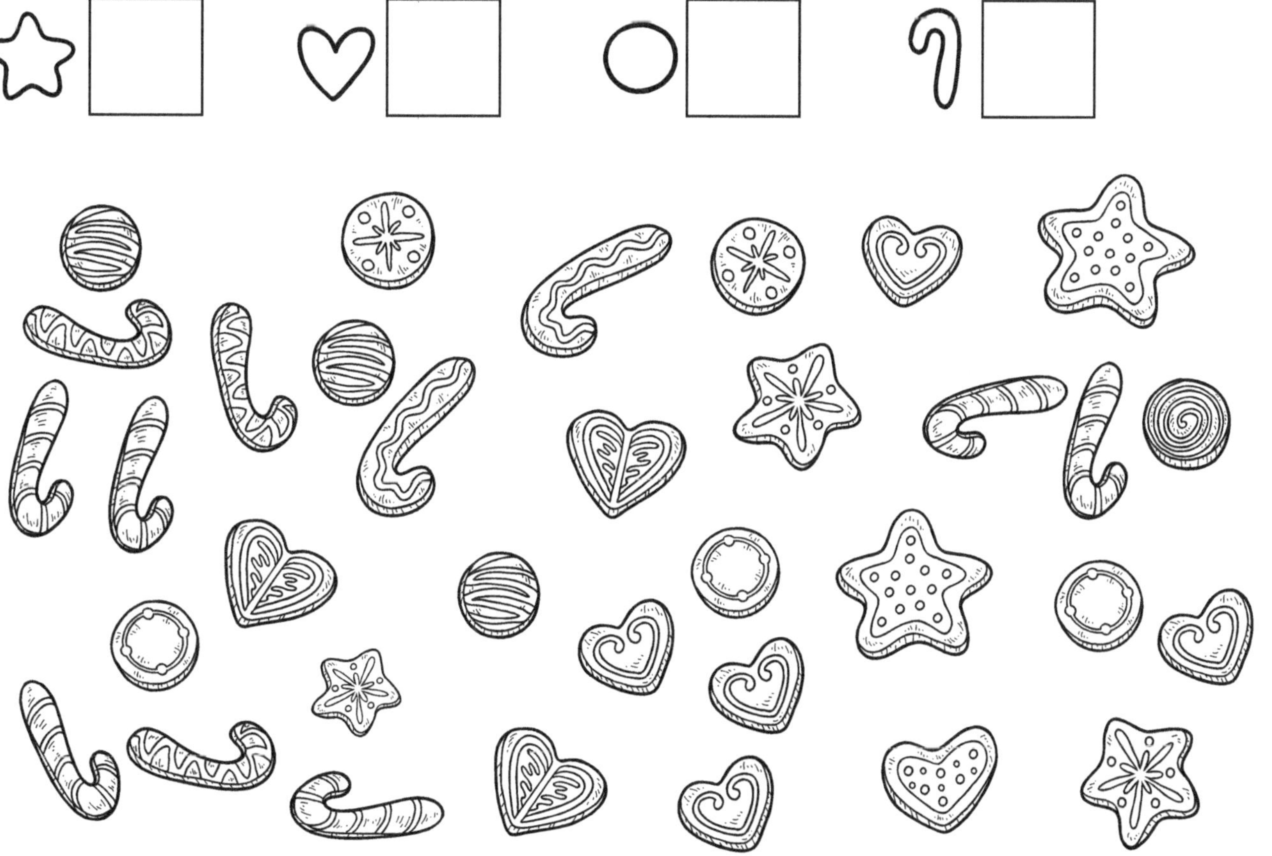

31. Dot to dot.

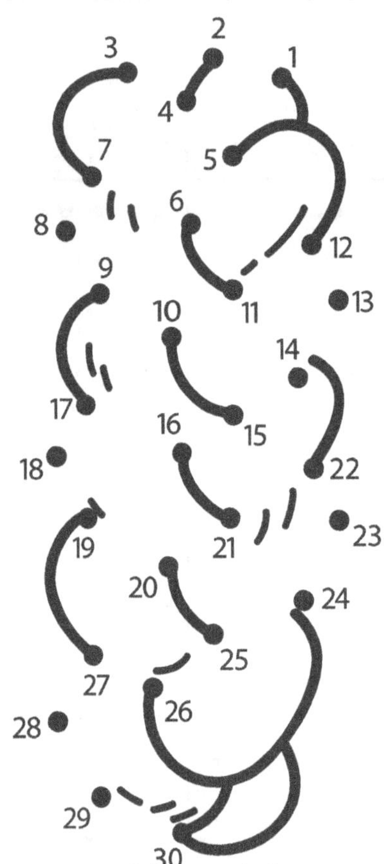

32. Read and remember, cover with your hand and write from memory.

20 40 60 80	
26 46 66 86	

33. Write down all the words that you know describing the word -Idea:

....

....

....

....

....

....

34. <, > or =

3.≤4   20...22
7....9   17....19
12....11   13....11
13....14   33....133
11.....10   111.....110
16....26   16....116
35....38   35...38

35. Matching game.

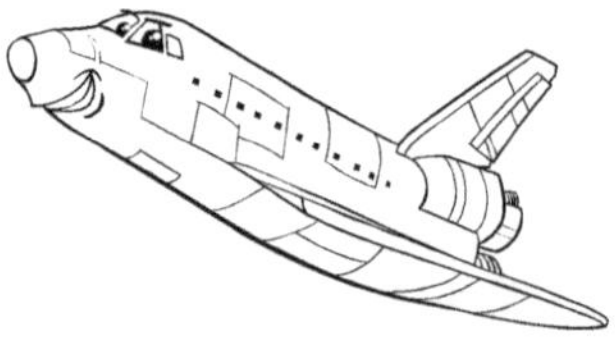

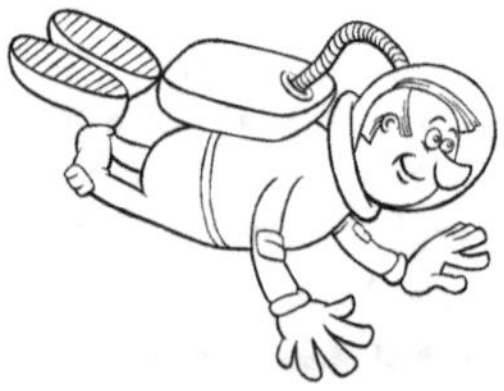

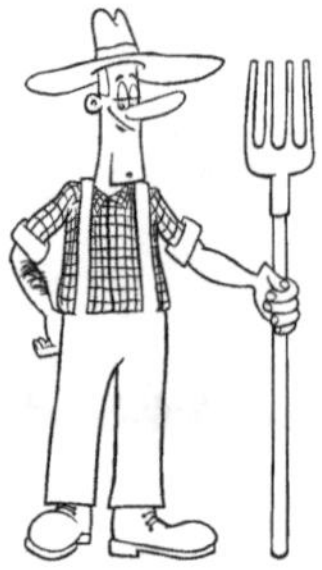

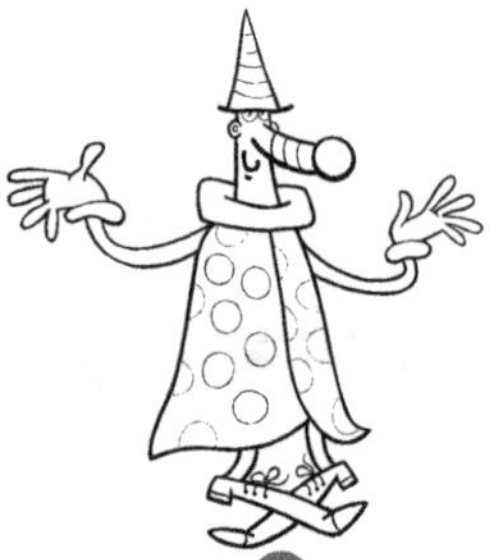

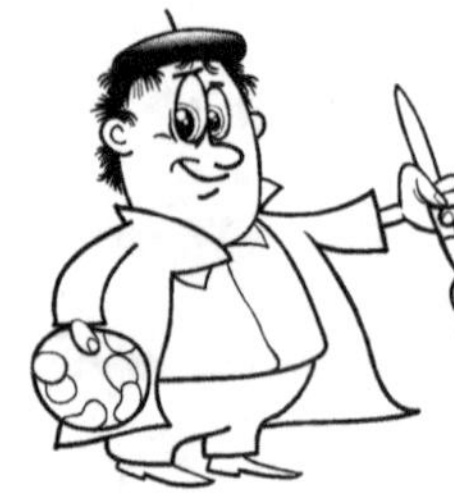

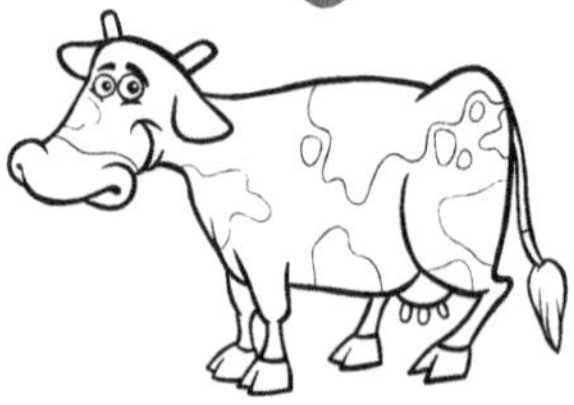

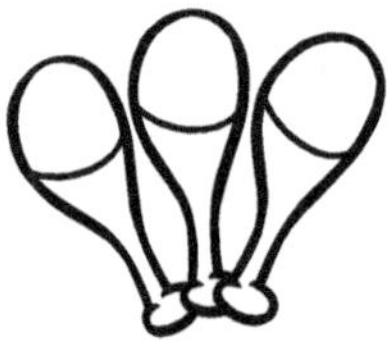

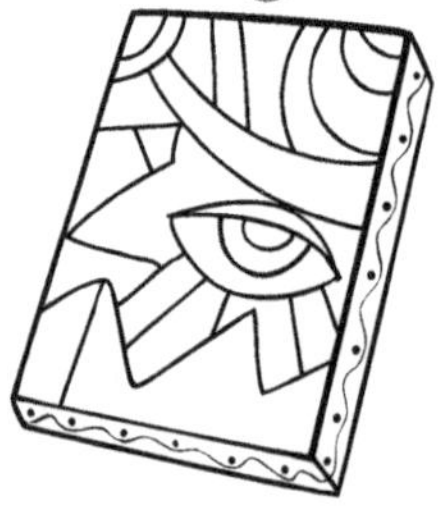

36. Copy the picture.

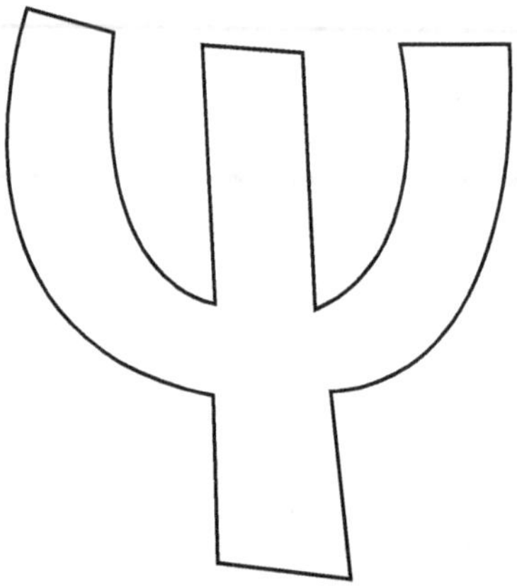

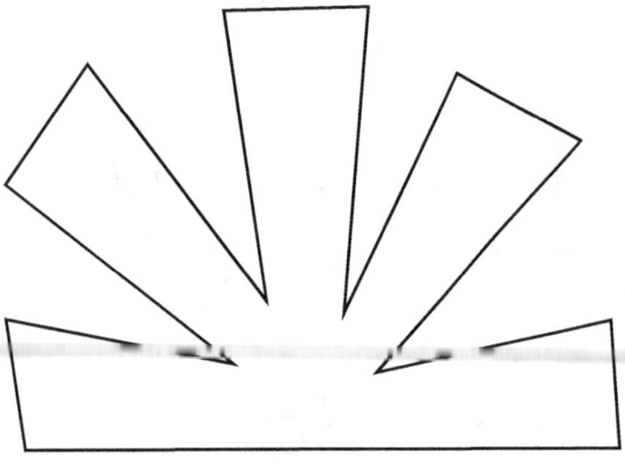

37. Dot to dot.

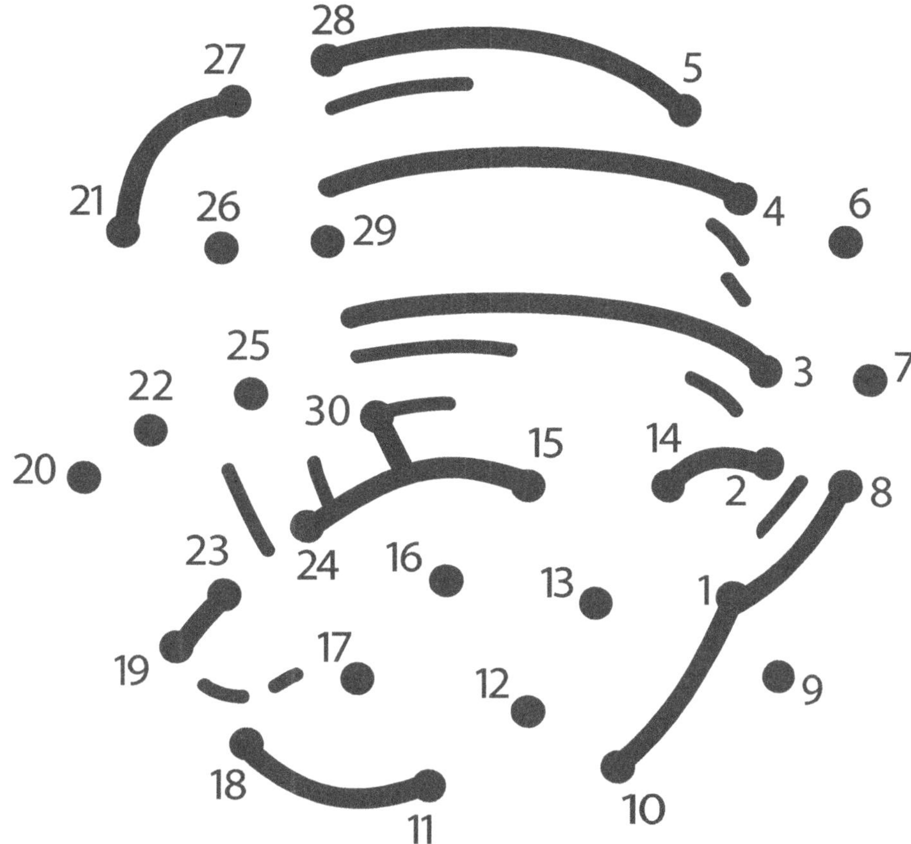

38. Counting game.

22+8=...   18-4=...
15+6=...   17-8=...
88+9=...   77-8=...
17+9=   16-7=
21+11=   11-8=
12+9=   12-9=
11+10=   11-5=

39. How many?

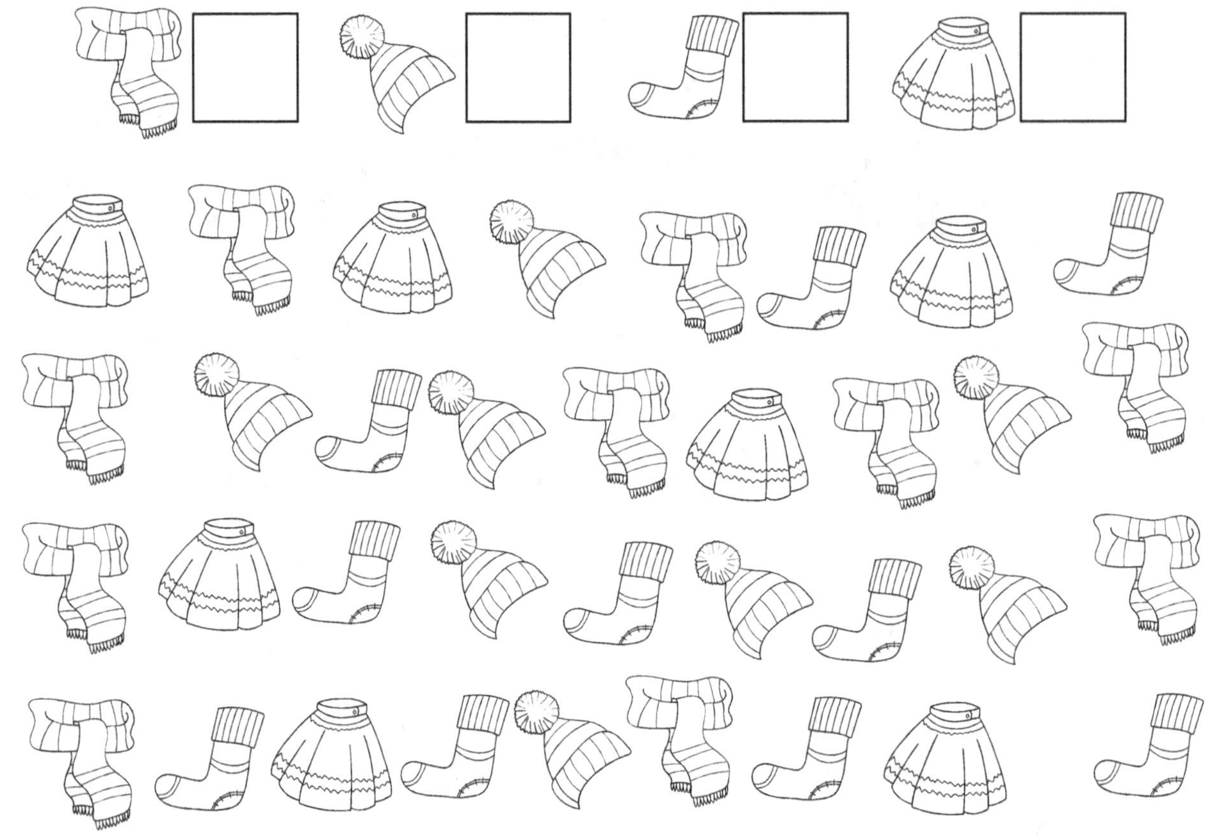

40. Mark kitchen tools.

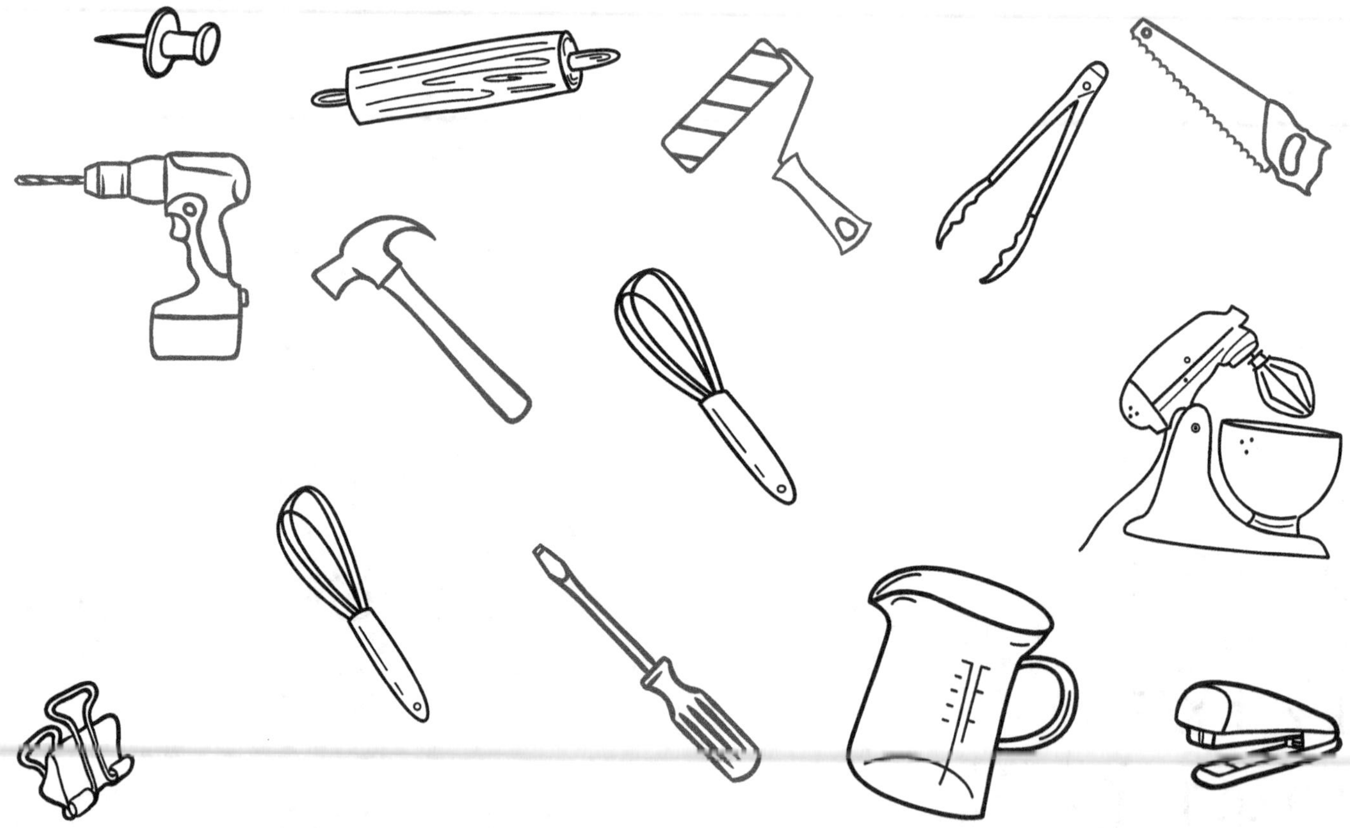

41. List as many words as possible from the category
Trees:

. . . .

. . . .

. . . .

. . . .

. . . .

. . . .

73. Write down what you see in the picture.

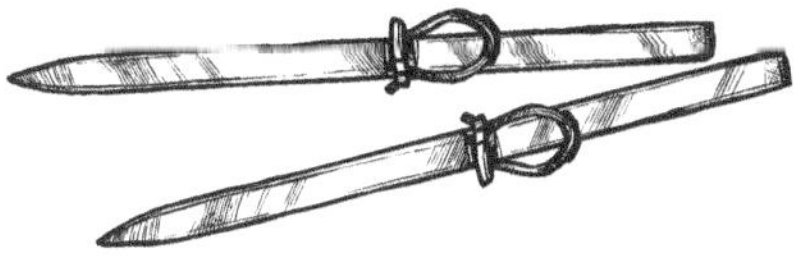

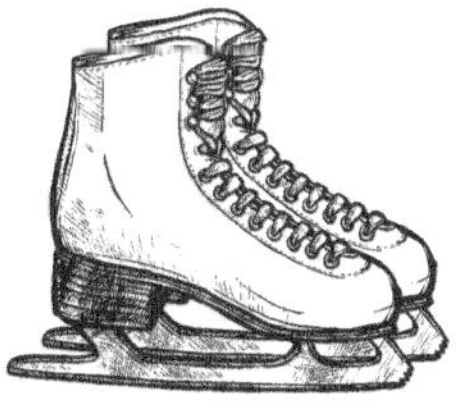

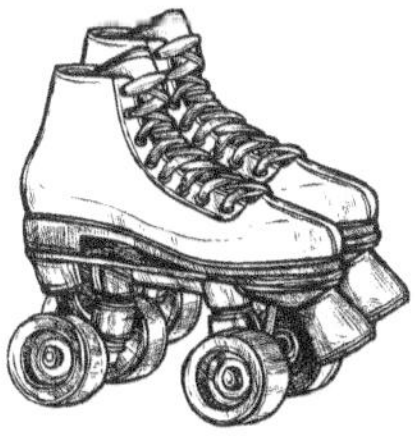

. . . .

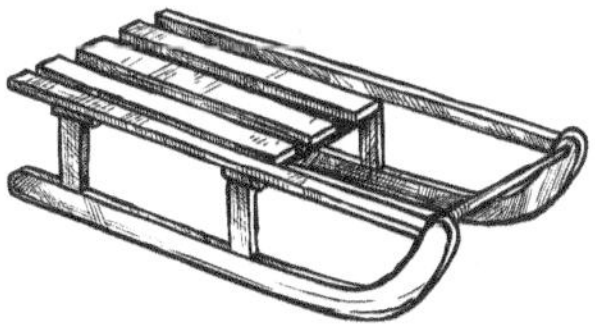

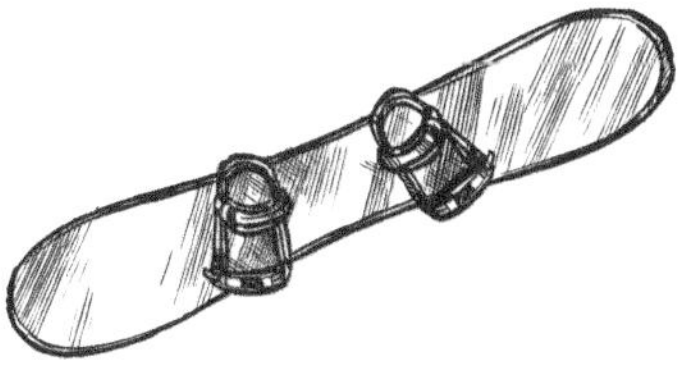

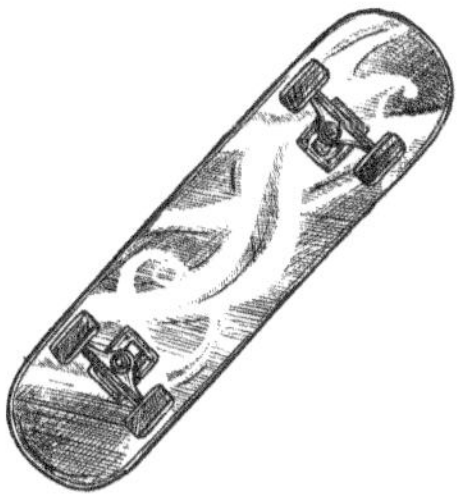

. . . .

43. Maze game.

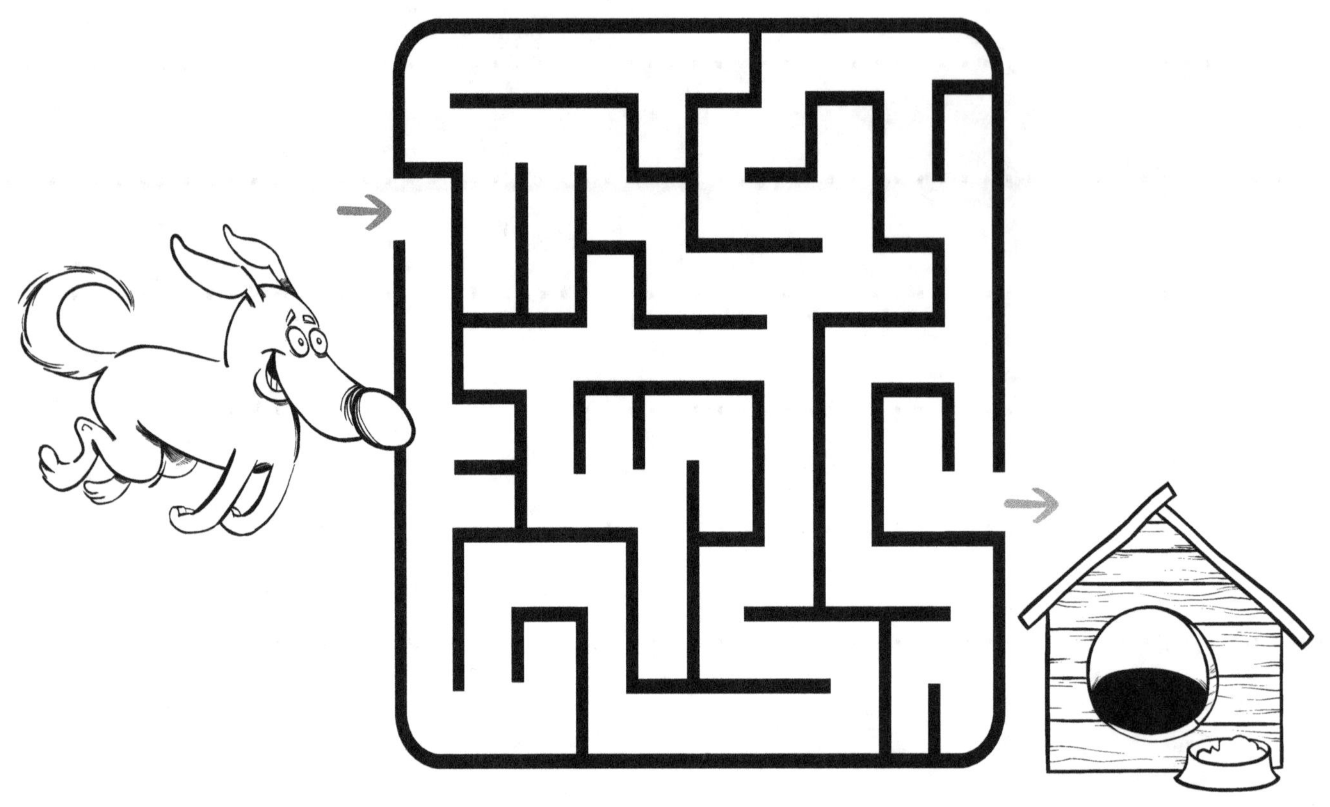

44. Describe your best vacation. Who did you spend this vacation with?

....

....

....

....

....

....

45. Word search puzzle.

D	M	V	T	E	N	T	R	L	C	I
I	N	U	C	Q	S	O	G	L	D	O
V	S	Y	H	X	E	W	Z	E	M	Y
I	A	J	J	P	A	E	O	J	O	D
N	I	L	A	H	S	L	T	Z	V	S
G	L	B	I	I	H	G	T	O	V	U
H	I	E	B	K	E	K	W	G	A	N
H	N	A	X	I	L	U	A	S	M	B
H	G	C	U	N	L	Y	V	N	F	A
P	A	H	B	G	M	L	E	D	D	T
L	C	Z	Y	V	E	P	D	W	N	H
N	C	P	O	M	F	X	F	A	N	E

BEACH
DIVING
FAN
HIKING
SAILING
SEASHELL
SUNBATHE
WAVE
TOWEL
TENT

46. Write down all the words that you know describing the word - Eyes:

....

....

....

....

....

47. Find 7 differences.

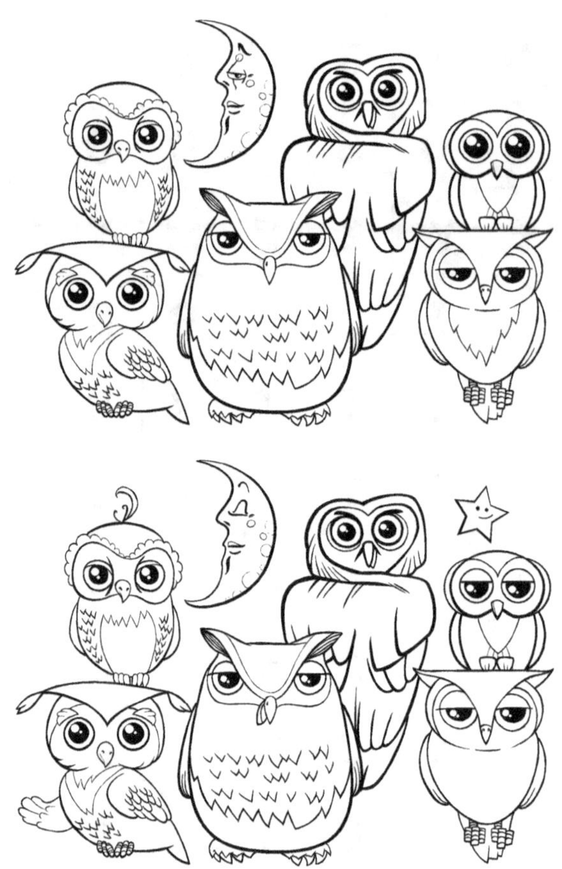

48. Read and remember, cover with your hand and write from memory.

3 33 63 93	
4 44 44	
4	

49. Name as many names starting with letter A as you can:

....

....

....

....

....

....

50. Read and remember, cover with your hand and write from memory.

spoon fork knife	
cooker fridge oven	

51. How many?

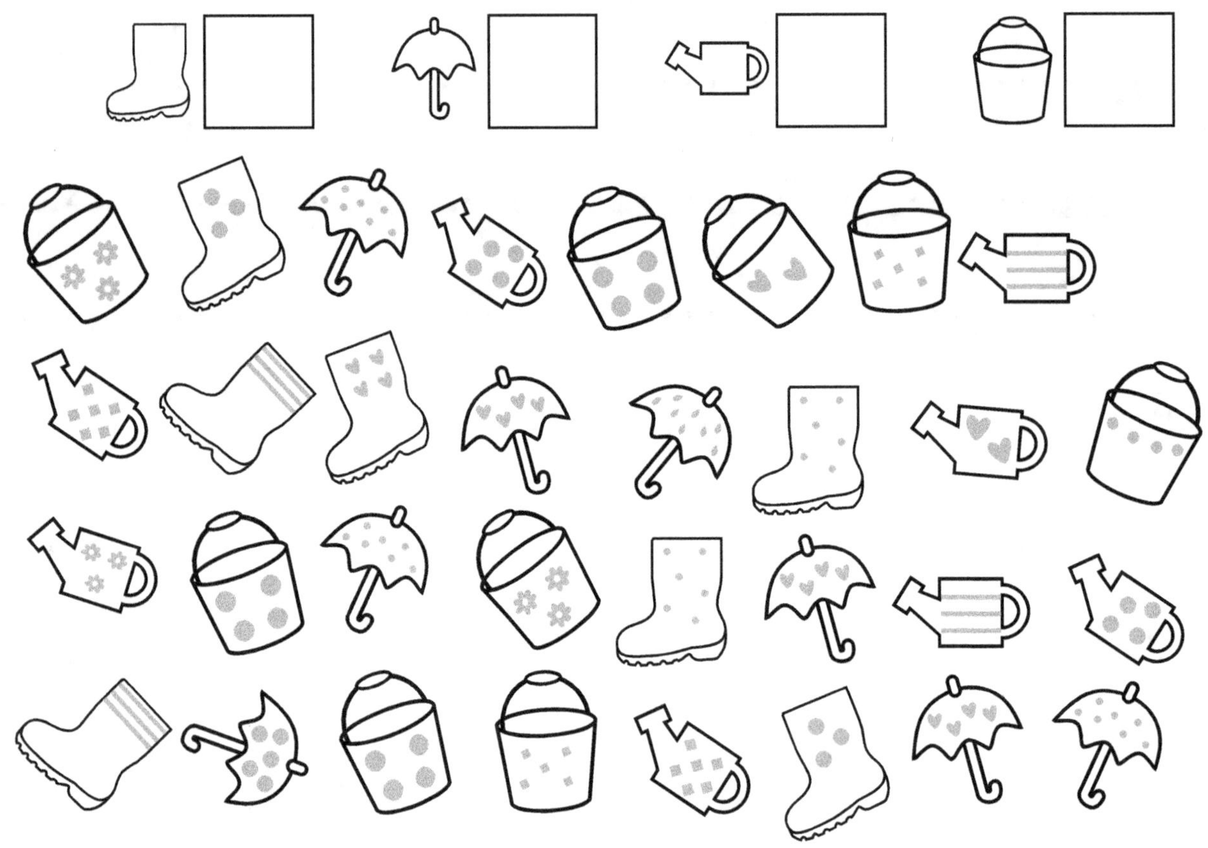

52. Find two the same picture

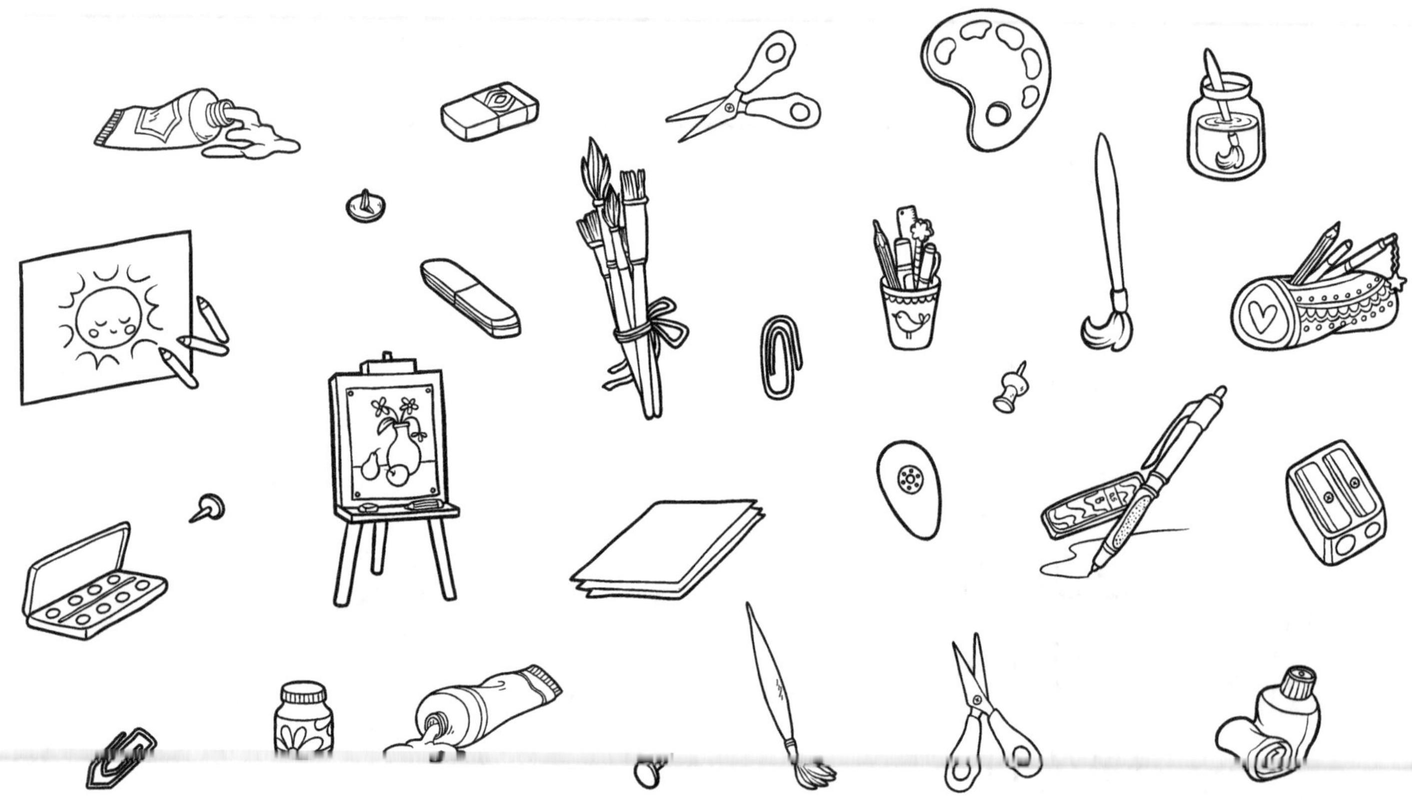

53. Find and circle every letter S.

S A S T D A R
F N A X L B Z
Z A B A D K A D E
Z A S A A S K A
A L C A S F Z

54. Dot to dot.

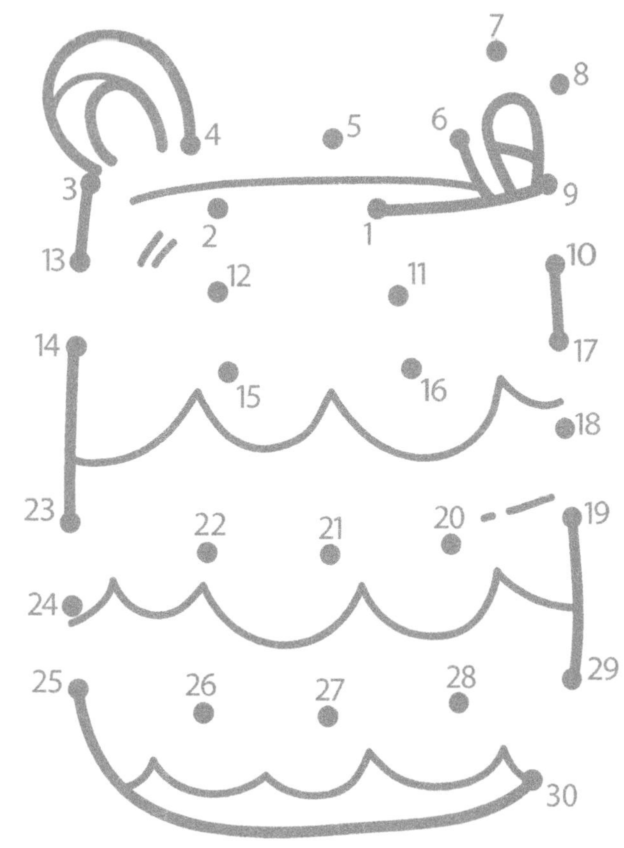

55. Write down what you see in the picture.

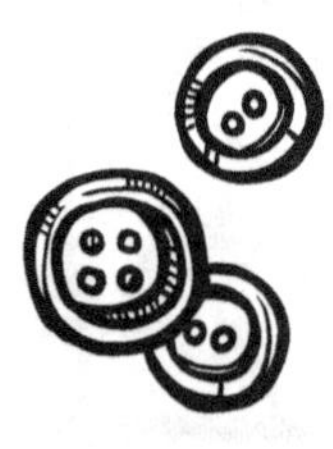

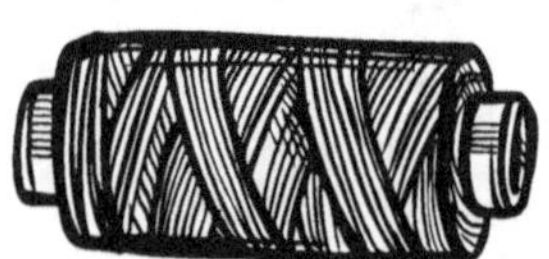

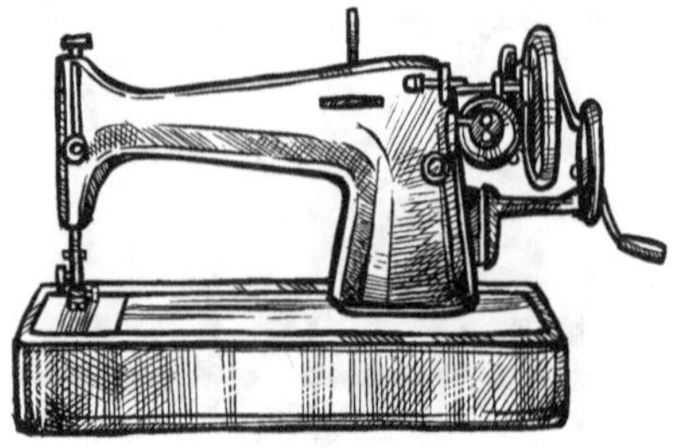

. . . .

. . . .

. . . .

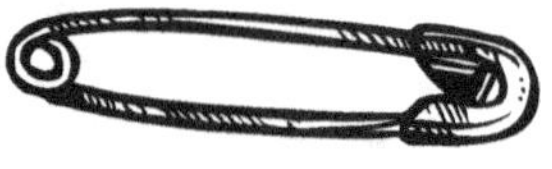

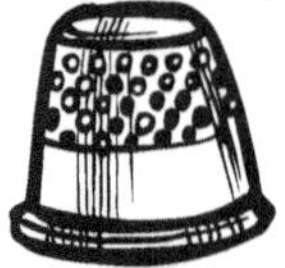

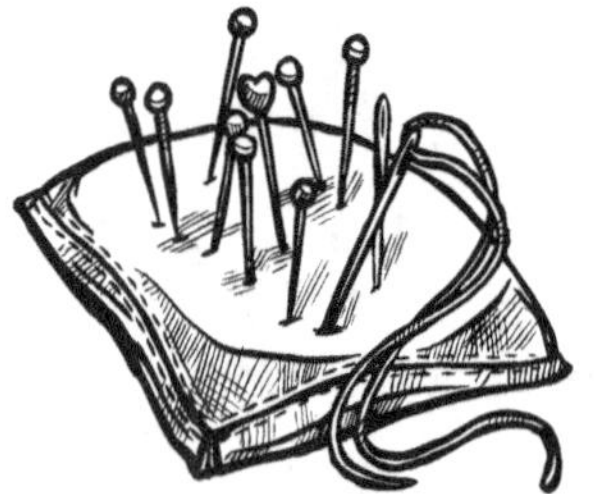

. . . .

. . . .

. . . .

56. Name as many soups as you can.

. . . .

. . . .

. . . .

. . . .

. . . .

. . . .

57. Matching game.

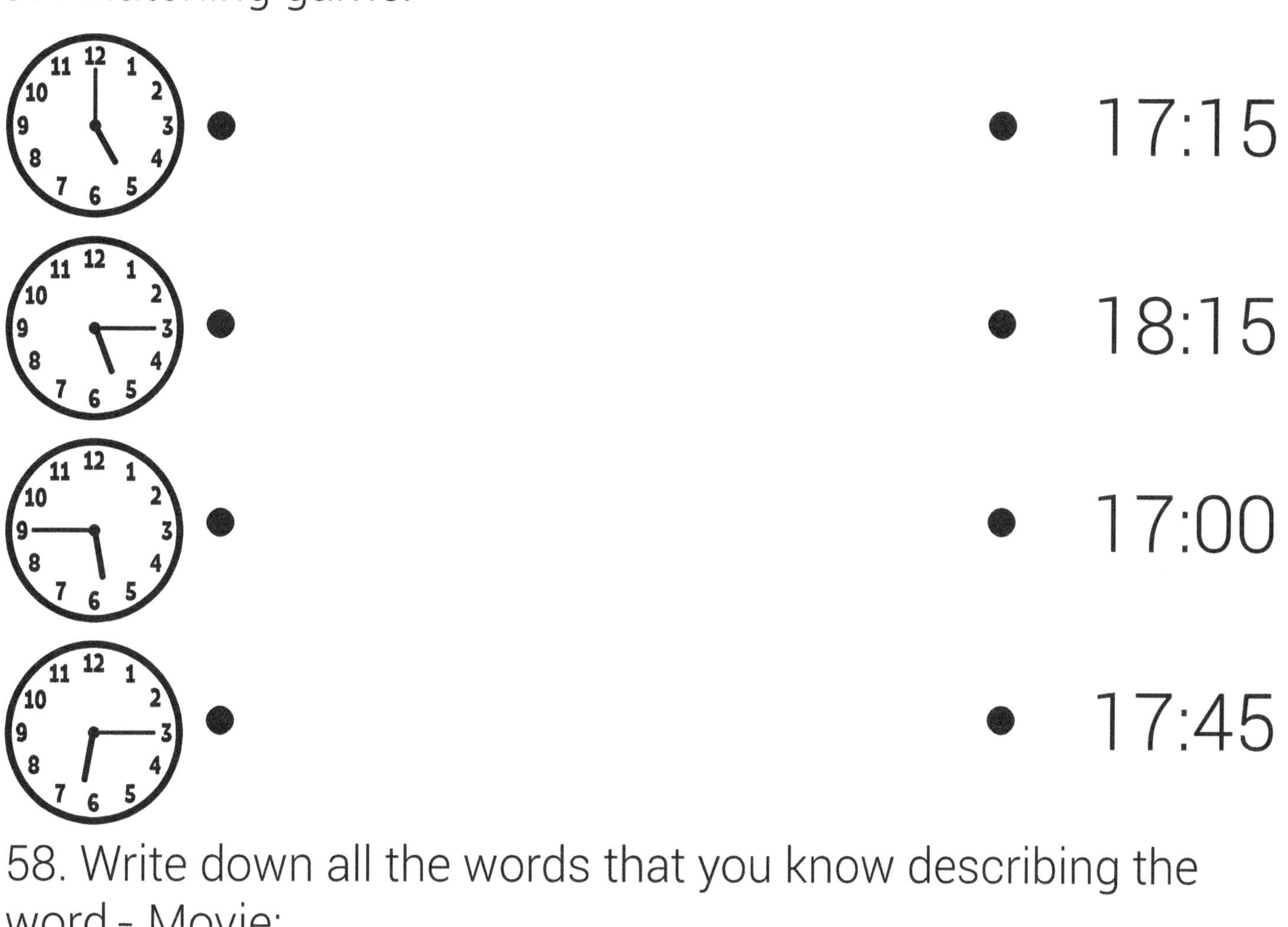

58. Write down all the words that you know describing the word - Movie:

....

....

....

....

....

....

59. Copy the picture.

60. Name as many names starting with letter S as you can.

61. Read and remember, cover with your hand and write from memory.

6 66 666 1666	
8 88 888 2888	

62. Find and circle every letter N.

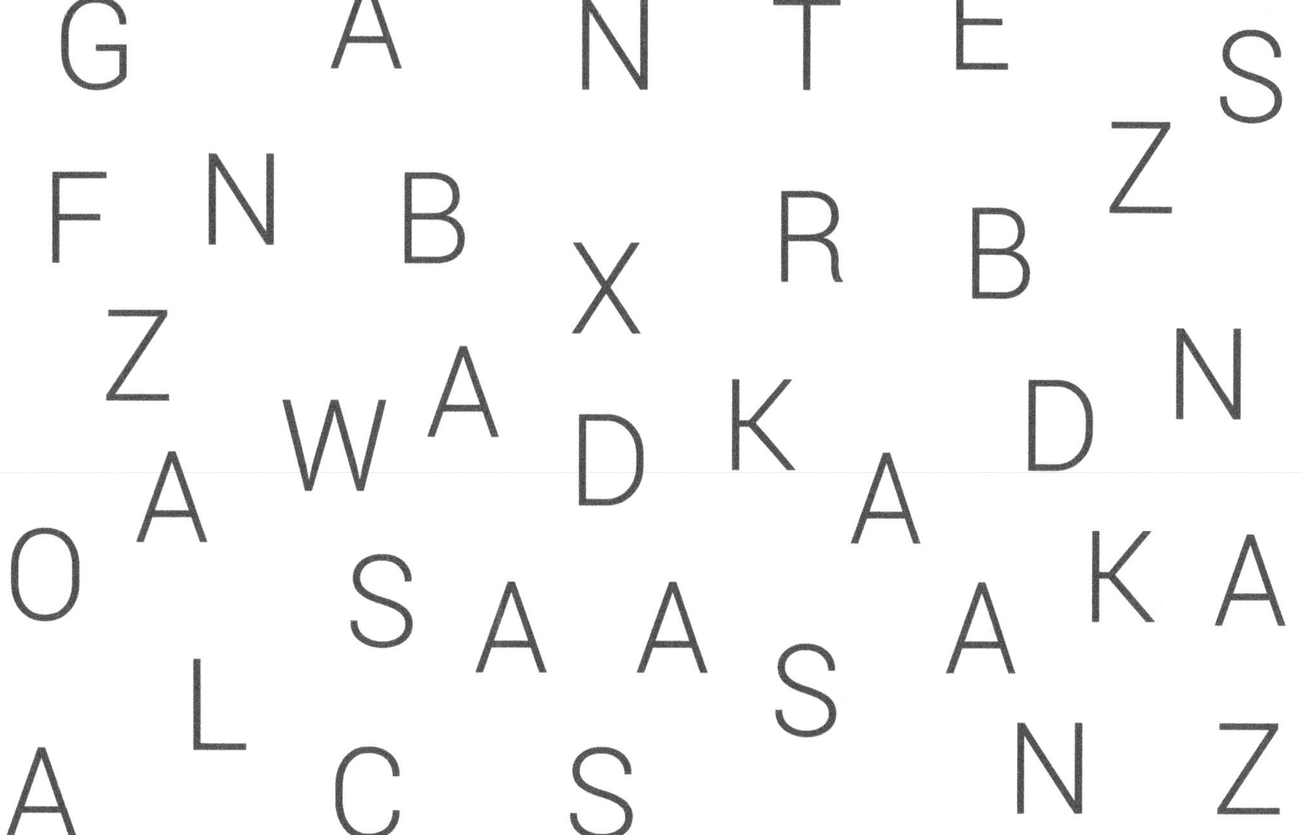

63. <, > or =

103...113	202...220
17....29	107....109
22....21	103....101
43....44	303....133
110.....101	101.....110
106....206	76....66
135....138	55....65

64. Write down places in which we buy medicine and breadstuff.

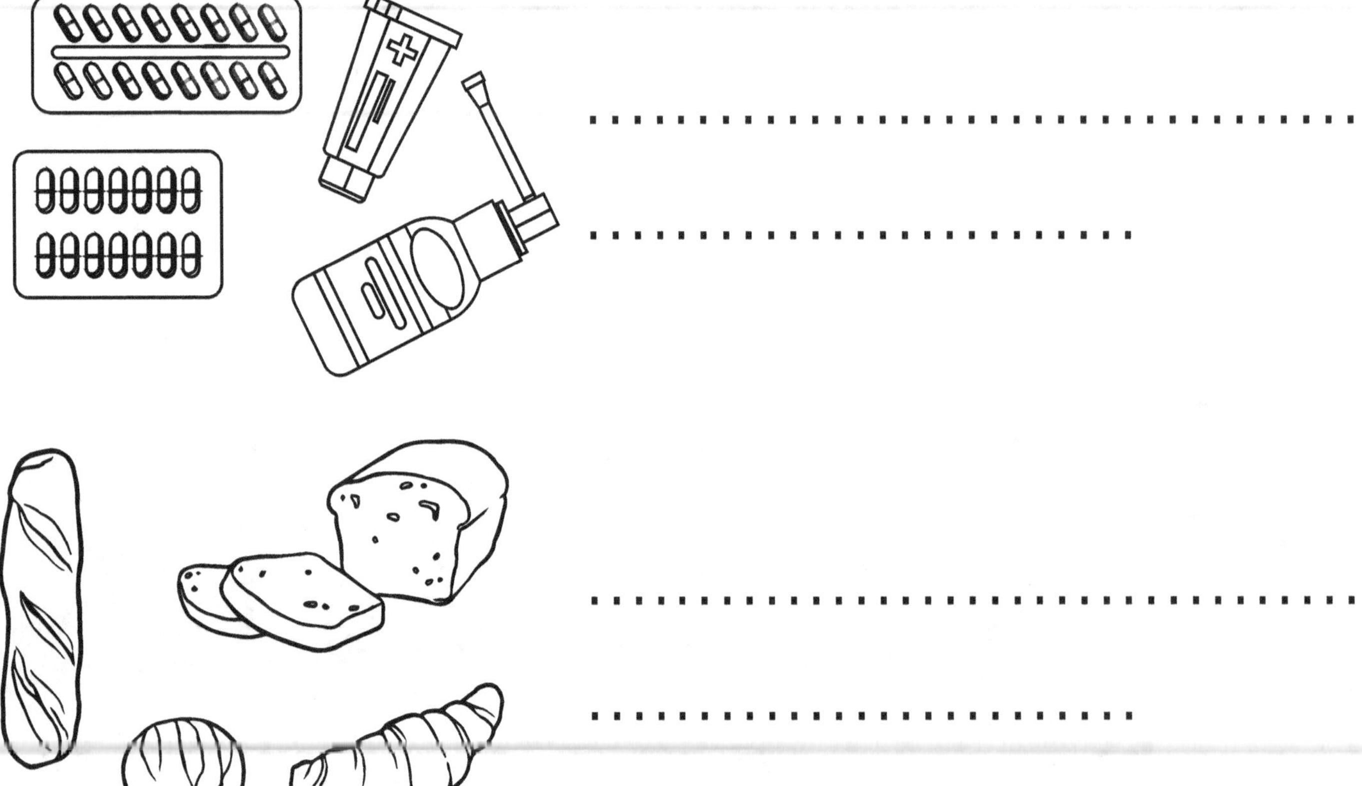

....

....

....

....

65. Copy the picture.

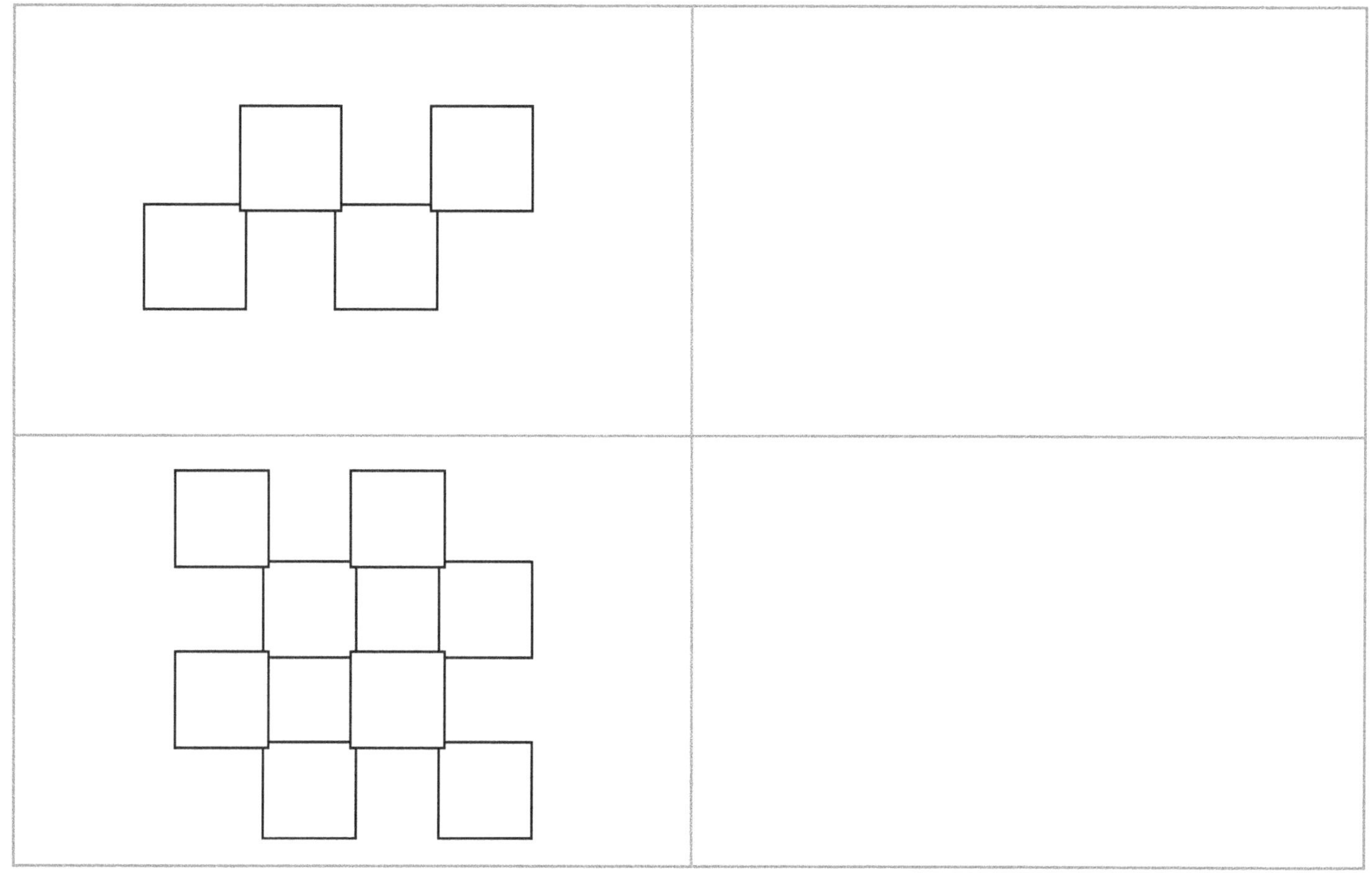

66. Find the numbers: 22.

12   32   22   92   222

22   42   622   522   22

32   322   22   82   22

42   72   62   22   122

52   92   102   272   22

22   92   22   22   52

67. Find the numbers: 16.

16   36   26   96   226

26   46   626   526   16

36   326   66   86   26

46   76   66   26   126

56   96   106   276   16

16   96   16   26   56

68. Name as many cold dishes as you can.

....

....

....

....

....

. . . Find the numbers: 16. ....

69. Name dairy food products.

. . . .

. . . .

. . . .

. . . .

. . . .

. . . .

70. Word search puzzle.

C	O	W	I	N	D	R	O	B	H	H
C	H	E	S	T	N	U	T	R	U	P
M	E	W	Q	N	Q	G	O	O	M	U
K	A	A	E	O	L	U	U	W	B	M
P	S	I	E	C	U	M	Y	N	R	P
J	A	C	O	A	T	V	O	F	E	K
G	U	S	Q	U	I	R	R	E	L	I
K	T	G	K	L	F	S	A	I	L	N
P	U	A	F	N	E	V	N	O	A	T
E	M	K	F	K	L	B	G	I	T	W
K	N	K	O	Q	T	G	E	J	F	S
Q	M	C	G	N	X	X	X	I	N	Y

PUMPKIN
SQUIRREL
CHESTNUT
FOG
UMBRELLA
COAT
AUTUMN
WIND
BROWN
ORANGE

71. Write down what you see in the picture.

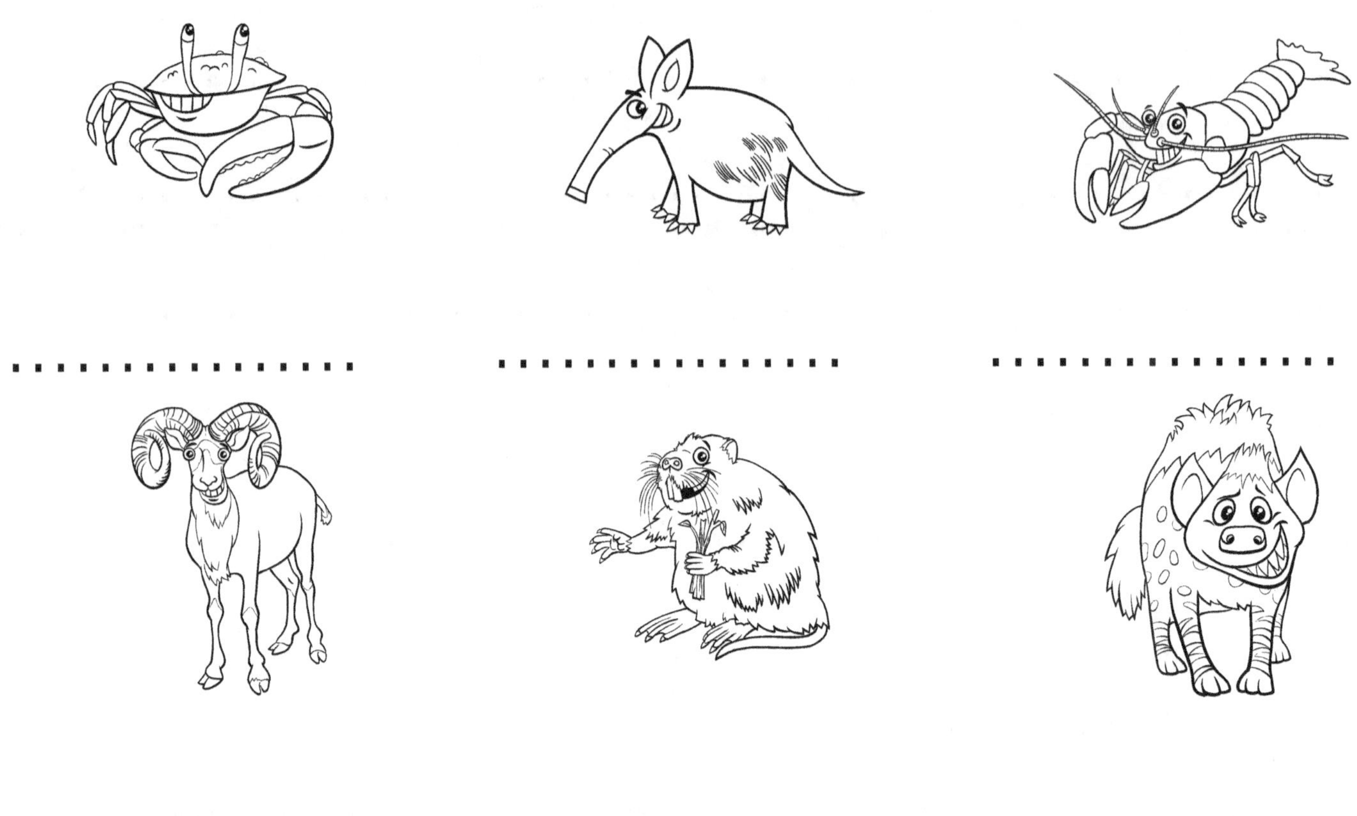

. . . .

. . . .

72. Copy the picture.

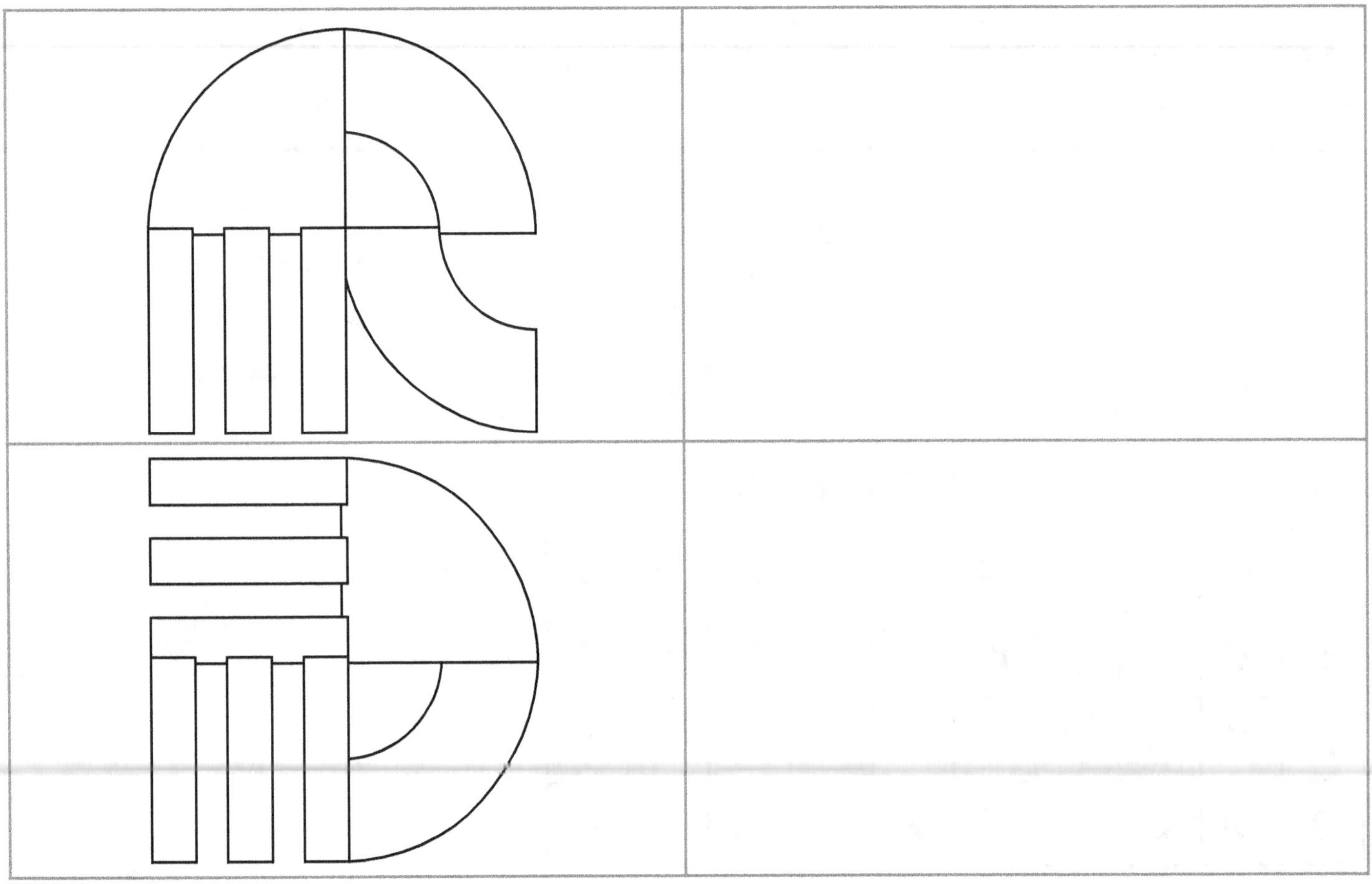

73. Mark the forest fruits and write down their names.

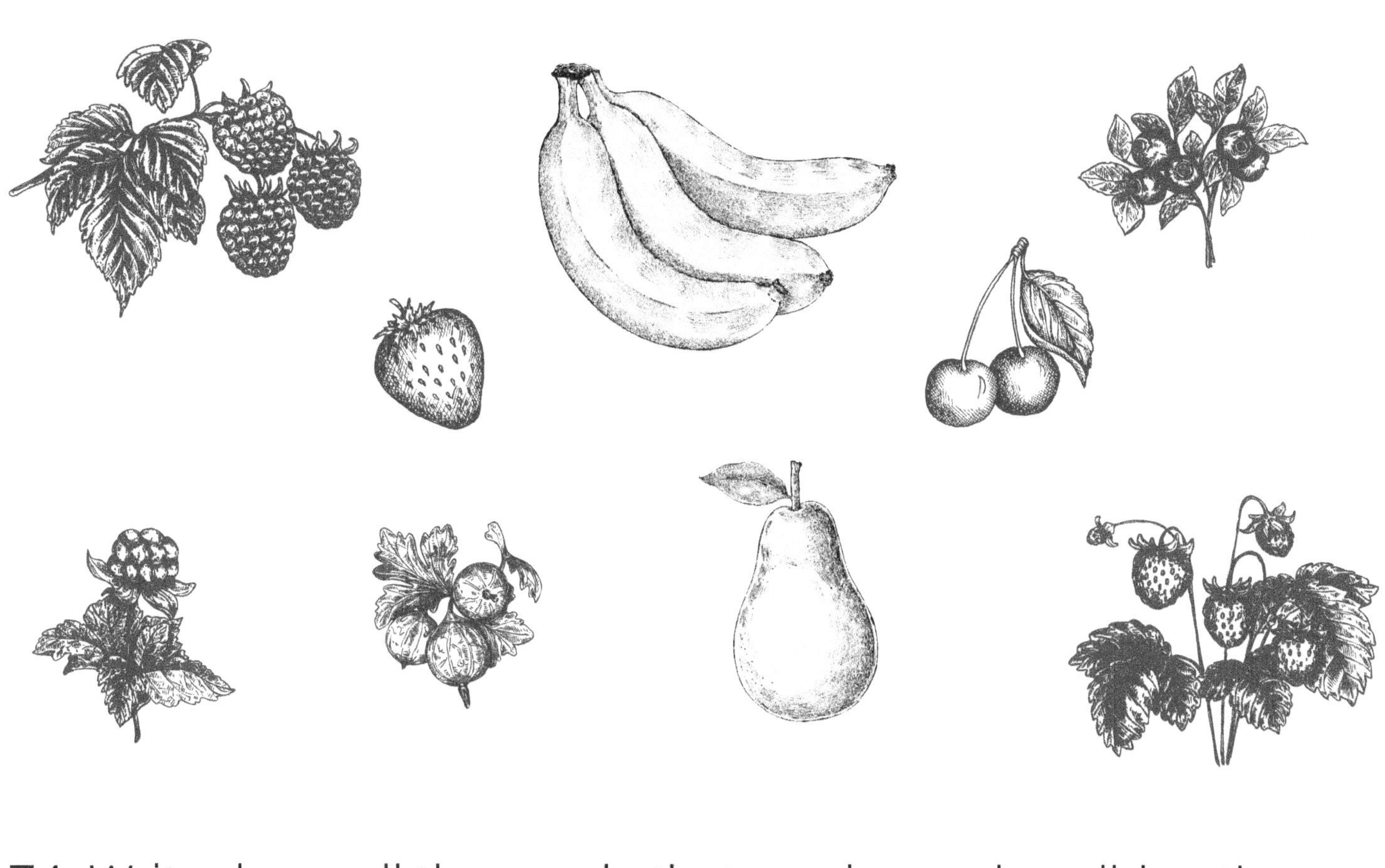

74. Write down all the words that you know describing the word - Flat:

....

....

....

....

....

....

75. Read and remember, cover with your hand and write from memory.

frying pan pot teapot	
cooker fridge oven	

76. List as many words as possible from the category
Fishes:

....

....

....

....

....

....

77. Match pairs.

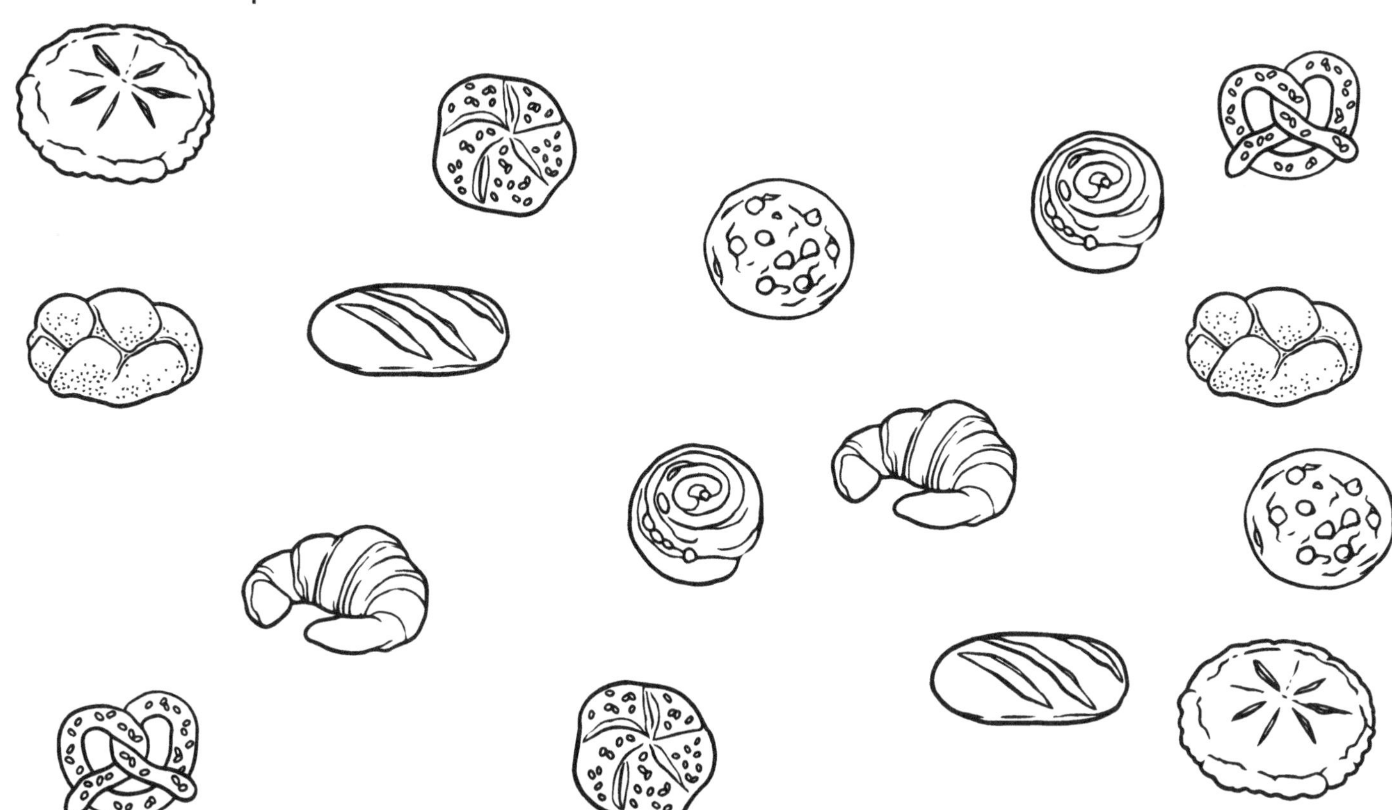

78. Matching game.

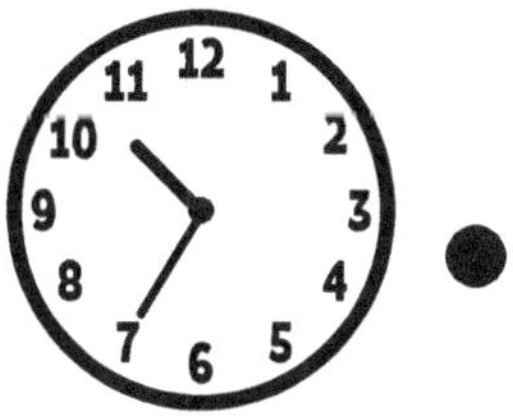

- 10:00
- 10:05 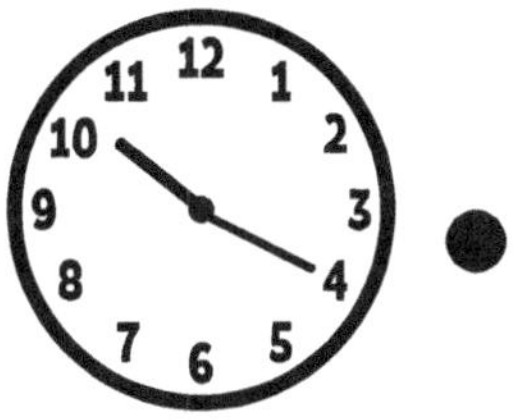
- 10:35 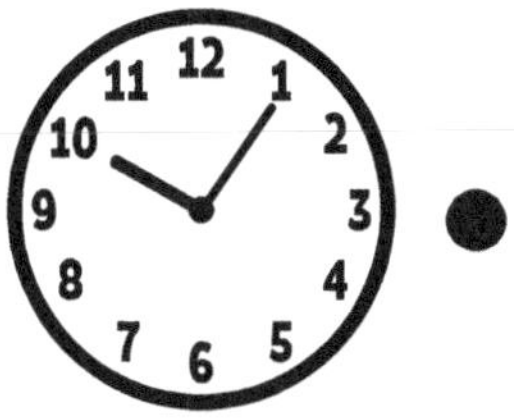
- 10:20

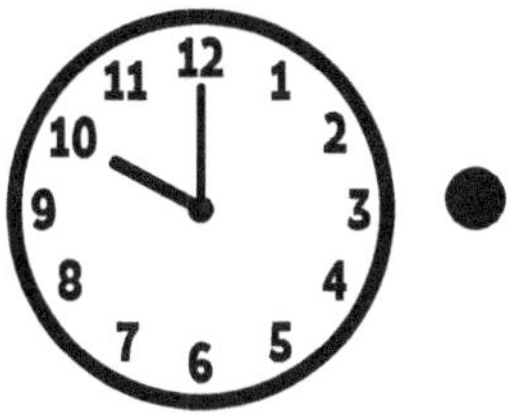

79. Name as many nouns starting with the letter A as you can:

....

....

....

....

....

....

80. Read and remember, cover with your hand and write from memory.

bath towel soap	
brush shampoo bangs	

DIFFICULT LEVEL

1. Dot to dot.

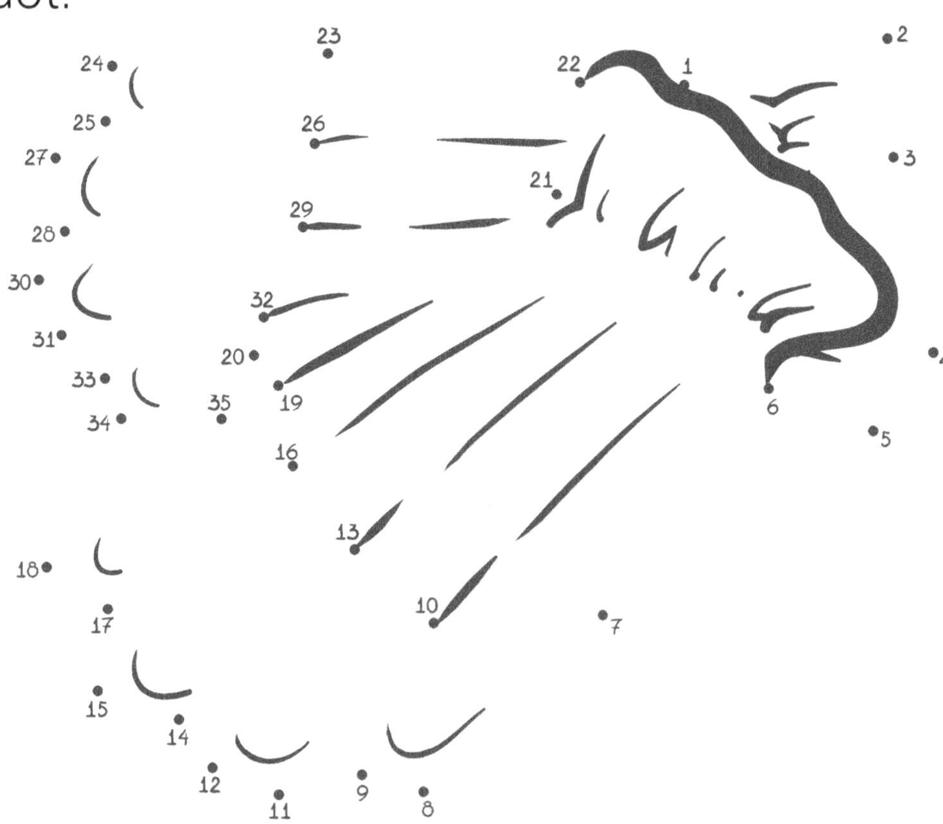

2. How many?

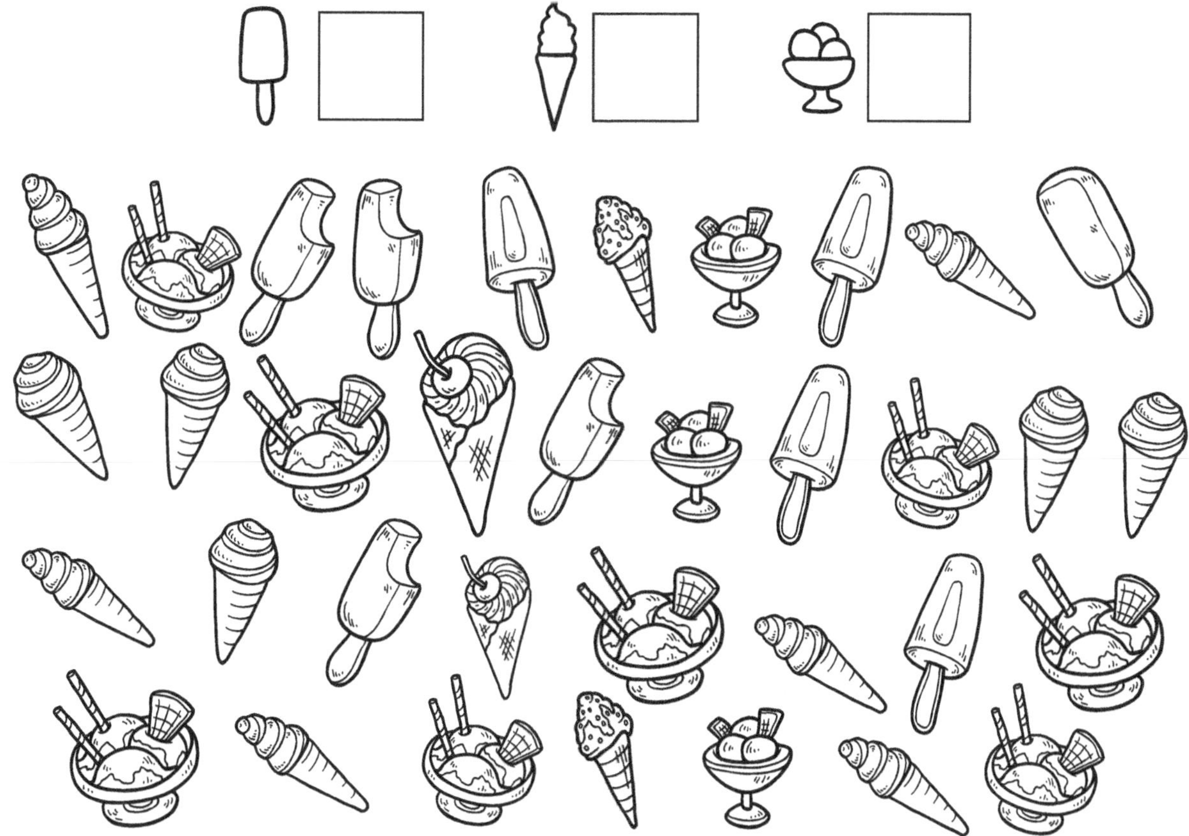

3. Write down as many types of footwear as you can.

....

....

....

....

....

....

4. Find 7 differences.

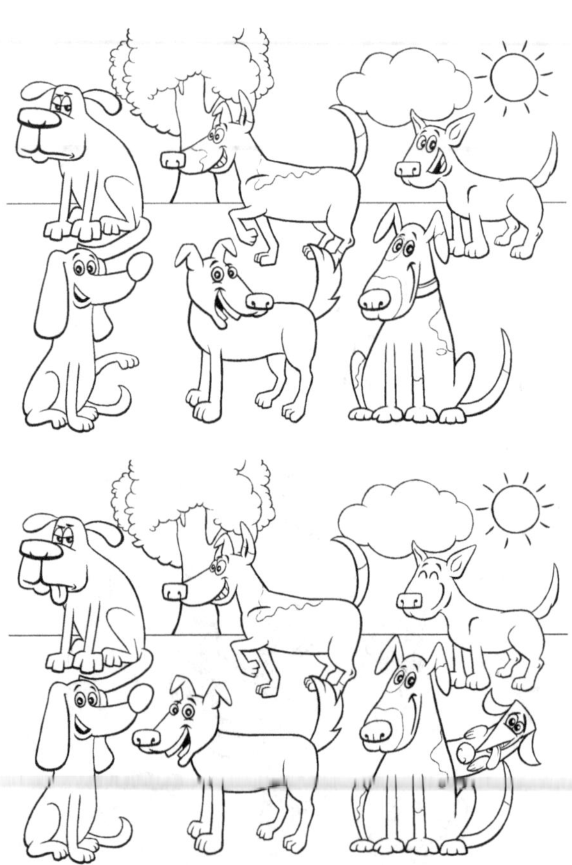

5. Name as many species of insects as you can.

....

....

....

....

....

6. Word search puzzle.

P	G	I	Y	Q	R	Q	C	P	N	I	W	K	V
I	J	W	E	I	Z	C	Y	C	L	I	N	G	N
E	Q	Z	B	W	U	O	O	W	R	C	U	I	N
H	O	R	S	E	R	A	C	I	N	G	M	L	G
S	F	G	X	V	D	X	Y	B	G	A	U	Q	D
S	J	O	B	D	F	D	T	S	G	E	L	U	I
A	Y	L	A	W	O	P	T	Z	J	R	B	K	V
I	M	F	S	F	Z	L	L	H	M	O	O	D	I
L	T	P	E	C	Q	G	H	C	B	B	X	U	N
I	K	C	B	M	Q	K	R	S	K	I	I	N	G
N	X	H	A	Y	M	S	S	Q	M	C	N	H	V
G	J	E	L	D	T	E	N	N	I	S	G	P	O
C	H	S	L	G	V	D	V	L	F	X	D	I	W
H	H	S	R	F	O	O	T	B	A	L	L	D	G

FOOTBALL
TENNIS
CYCLING
AEROBICS
BASEBALL
BOXING
CHESS
DIVING
GOLF
HORSERACING
SAILING
SKIING

7. Find and circle the letters db.

db   dd   db   dd
            bb   dd
bb   db   bd   db
         bd
      bd   db
bd   bd
      db   bb
dd   bd   bb

8. Name as many spices as you can.

....

....

....

....

....

9. List as many words as possible from the category
Herbs:

....

....

....

....

....

....

10. Write down all the words that you know describing the
word - Pen:

....

....

....

....

....

11. What does not fit?

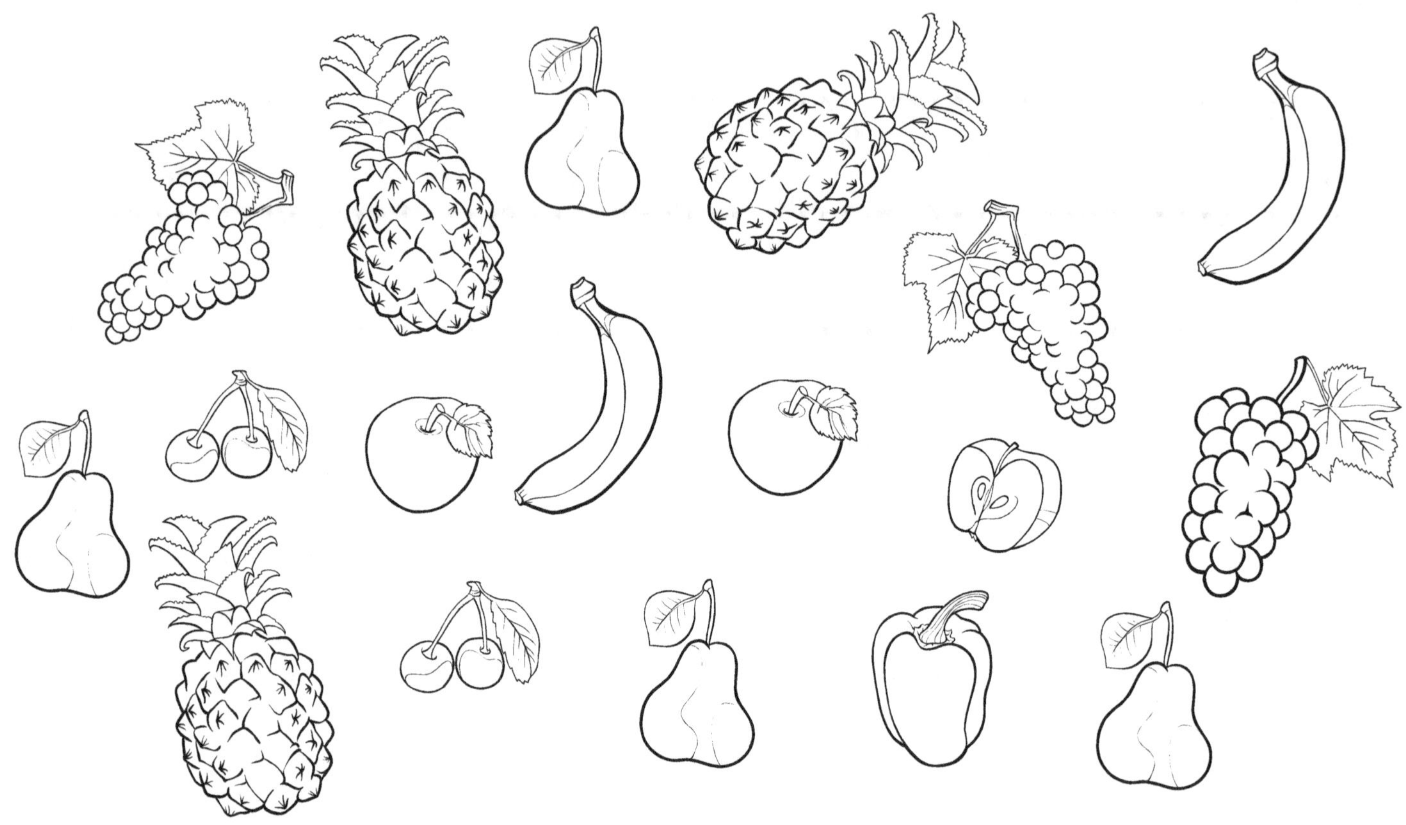

12. Counting game.

9+6=...   23+6=...
6+6=...   35+5=...
19+9=...   28+7=...
7+9=...   57+9=...
31+11=...   41+11=...
12+17=...   82+9=...
31+12=...   81+12=...

13. Dot to dot.

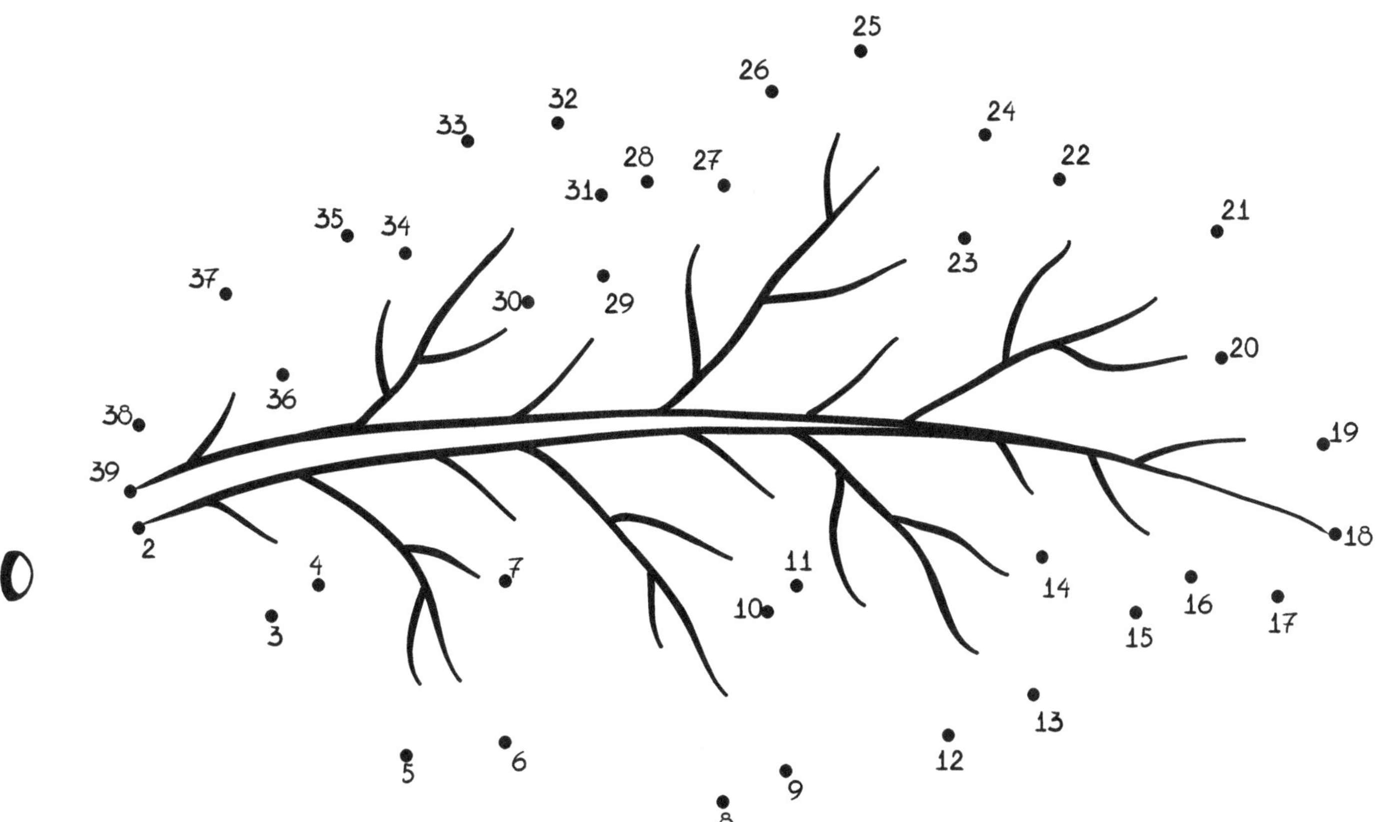

14. Read and remember, cover with your hand and write from memory.

3344 4455 5566	
2222 3222 4222	

15. Maze game.

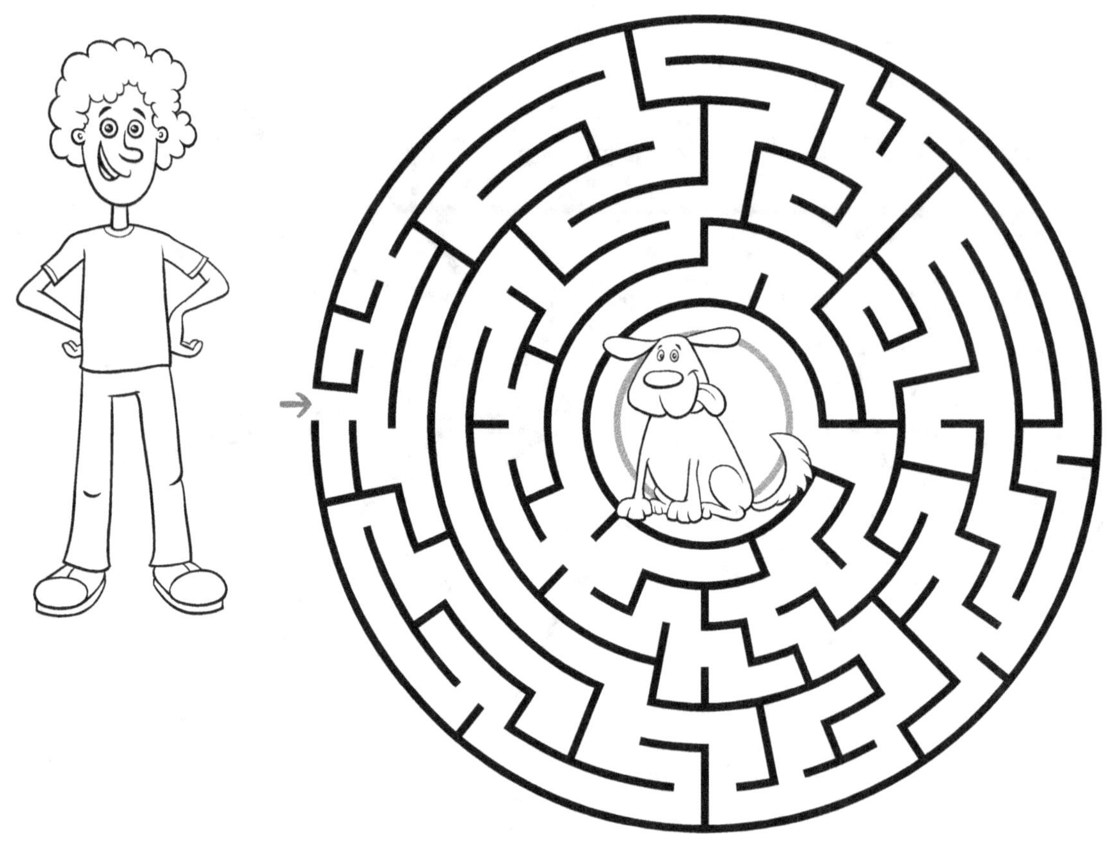

16. Copy the picture.

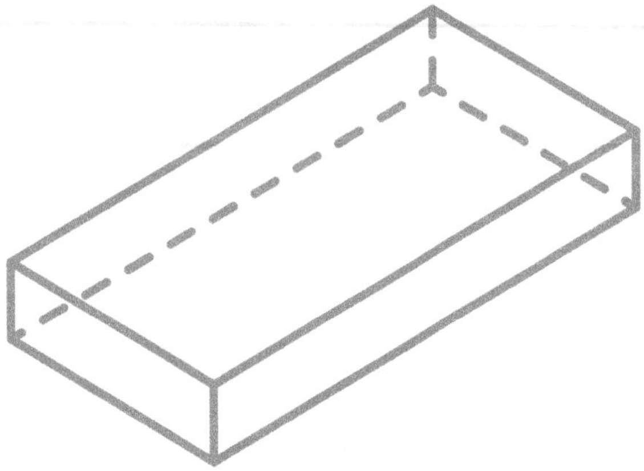

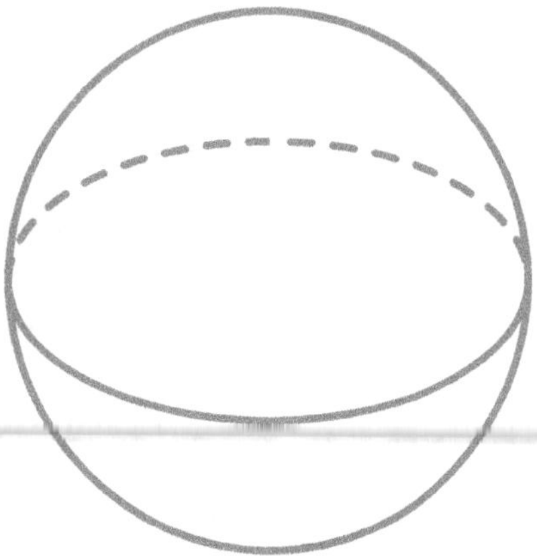

17. Write down what you see in the picture.

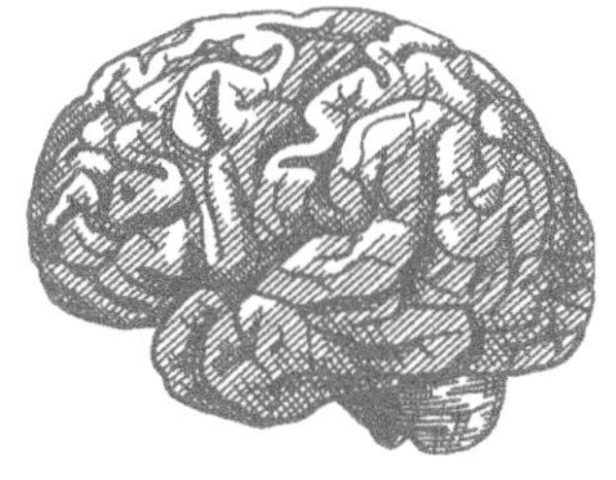   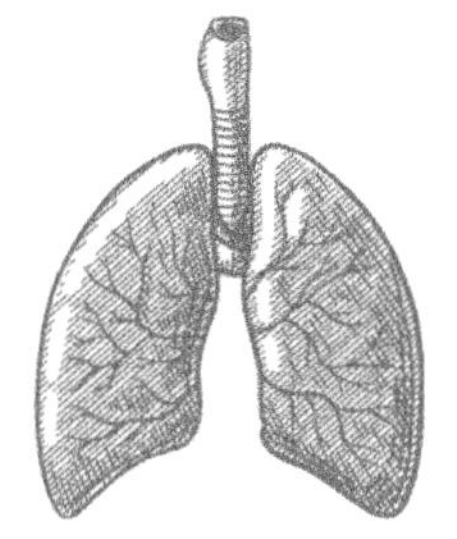   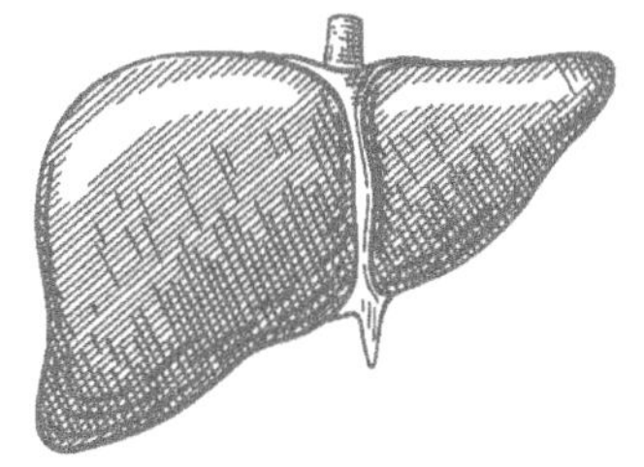

. . . .

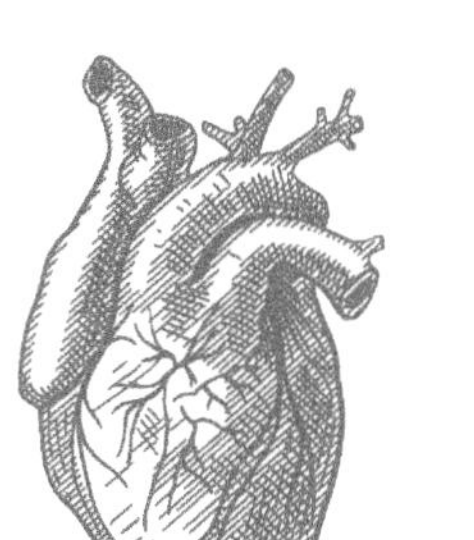   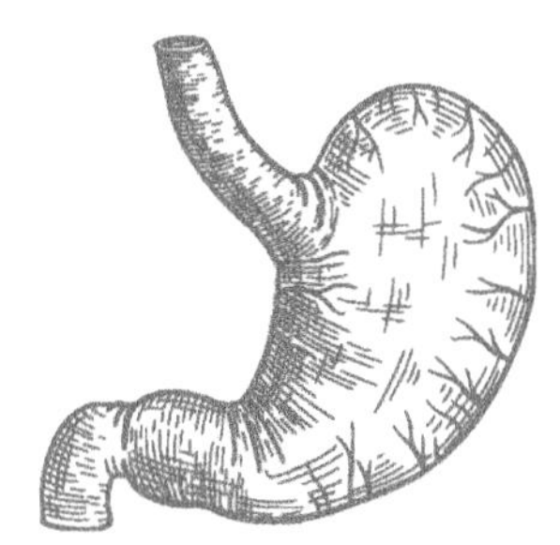   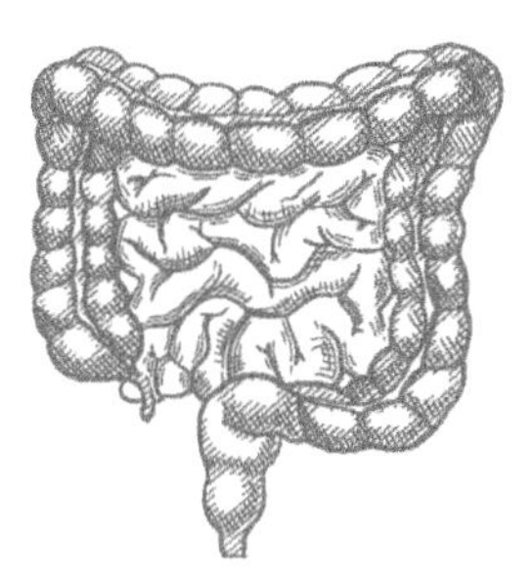

. . . .

18. How many?

19. What does not fit?

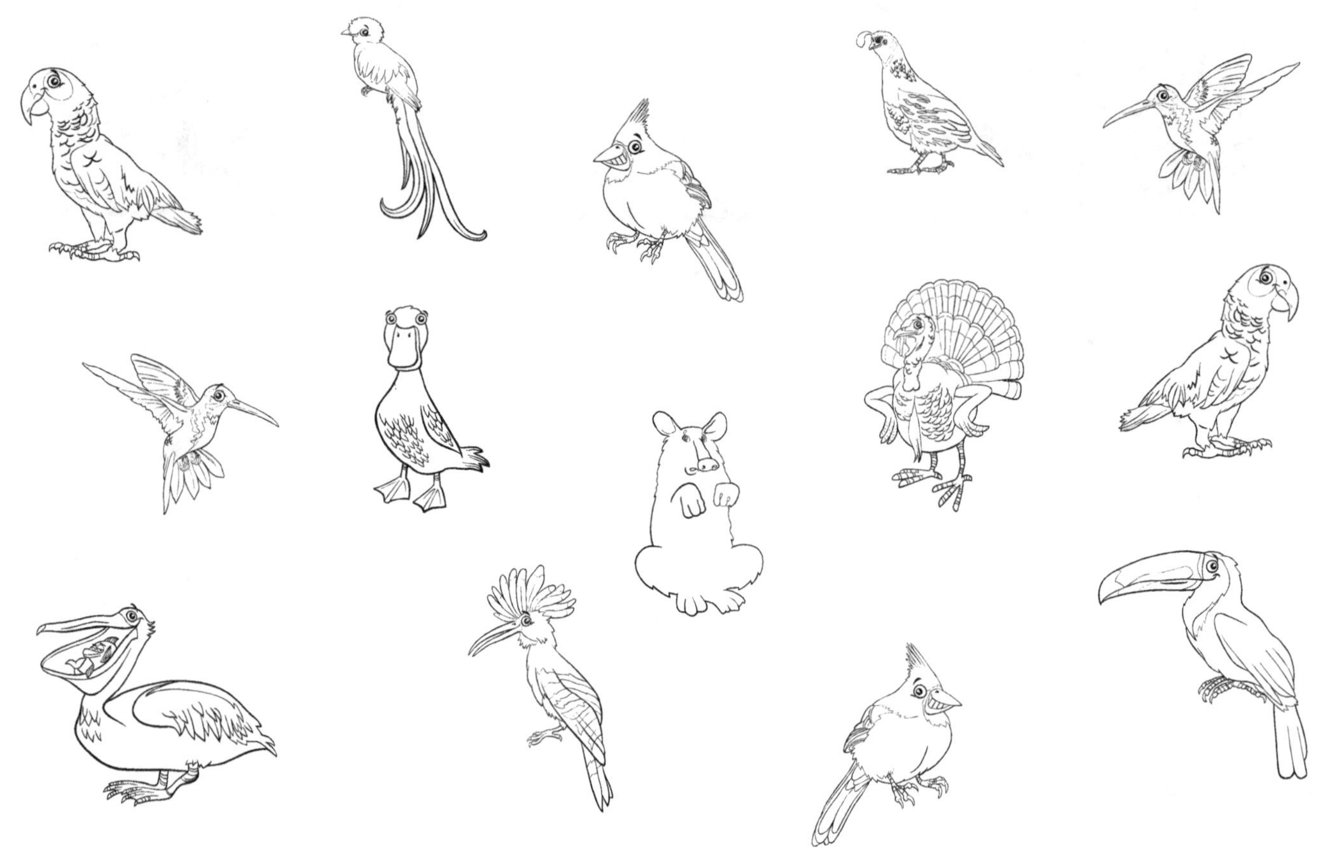

20. What are the synonyms for the words:

Party	Car
....	....
....	....
....	....
....	....
....	....

21. Counting game.

18-6=...	38-9=...
17-5=...	37-8=...
18-4=...	28-8=...
29-7=	76-7=
51-6=	81-6=
22-7=	42-7=
81-5=	31-5=

22. List as many words as possible from the category
Diseases:

....

....

....

....

....

23. Write down the names of the doctors treating parts of the body shown below.

. . . .

. . . .

. . . .

24. Write down all the words that you know describing the word - Apple:

. . . .

. . . .

. . . .

. . . .

. . . .

. . . .

25. Find 8 differences.

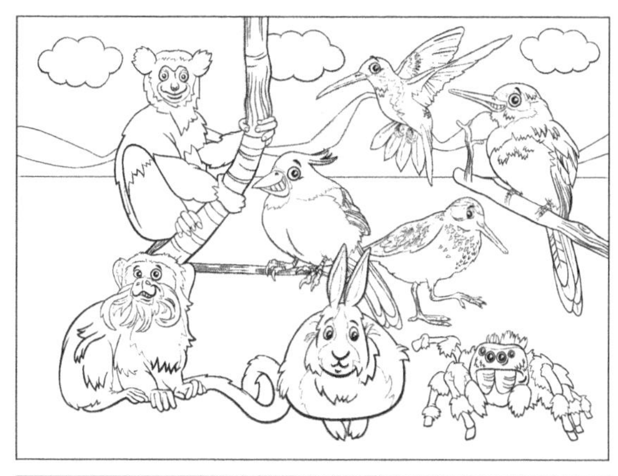

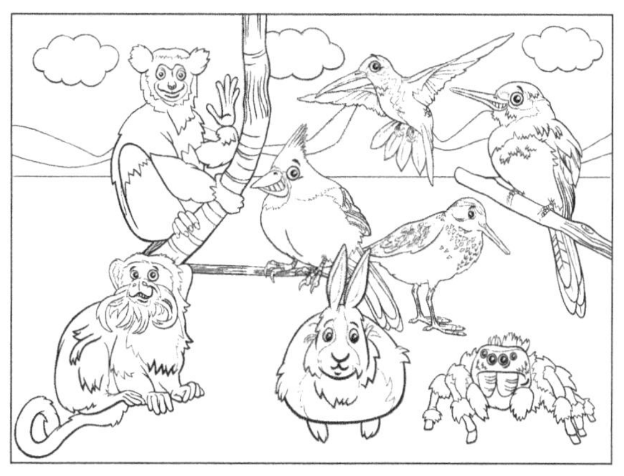

26. <, > or =

114...115

177....107

222....221

403....444

510.....501

109....106

1035....135

402...420

307....308

109....1009

133....1033

201.....210

76....67

505....565

27. Word search puzzle.

R	D	W	R	I	D	H	T	D	P	E	N	D	B
Y	R	B	V	Z	R	E	A	G	A	B	N	Y	H
S	I	J	Z	N	J	N	C	B	I	Y	U	P	H
S	V	V	P	G	U	K	A	V	N	M	R	V	B
D	E	I	H	D	D	T	R	K	T	U	S	L	X
Z	R	O	G	F	G	E	D	G	E	S	E	L	U
D	O	L	Z	R	E	D	I	J	R	I	T	T	S
I	T	I	D	S	O	W	O	J	E	C	E	N	P
R	B	N	E	I	E	G	L	S	P	I	A	N	M
E	C	I	N	N	J	G	O	I	A	A	C	S	L
C	J	S	T	G	Q	Z	G	X	B	N	H	N	Q
T	H	T	I	E	P	I	I	I	C	L	E	R	K
O	T	N	S	R	A	Q	S	J	X	A	R	R	X
R	M	Q	T	C	O	P	T	C	N	M	E	G	F

TEACHER
DENTIST
NURSE
CARDIOLOGIST
VIOLINIST
DIRECTOR
MUSICIAN
PAINTER
SINGER
JUDGE
CLERK
DRIVER

28. Name the countries of Asia.

....

....

....

....

....

....

29. What are the synonyms for the words:

House	Child
. . . .	. . . .
. . . .	. . . .
. . . .	. . . .
. . . .	. . . .
. . . .	. . . .

30. How many?

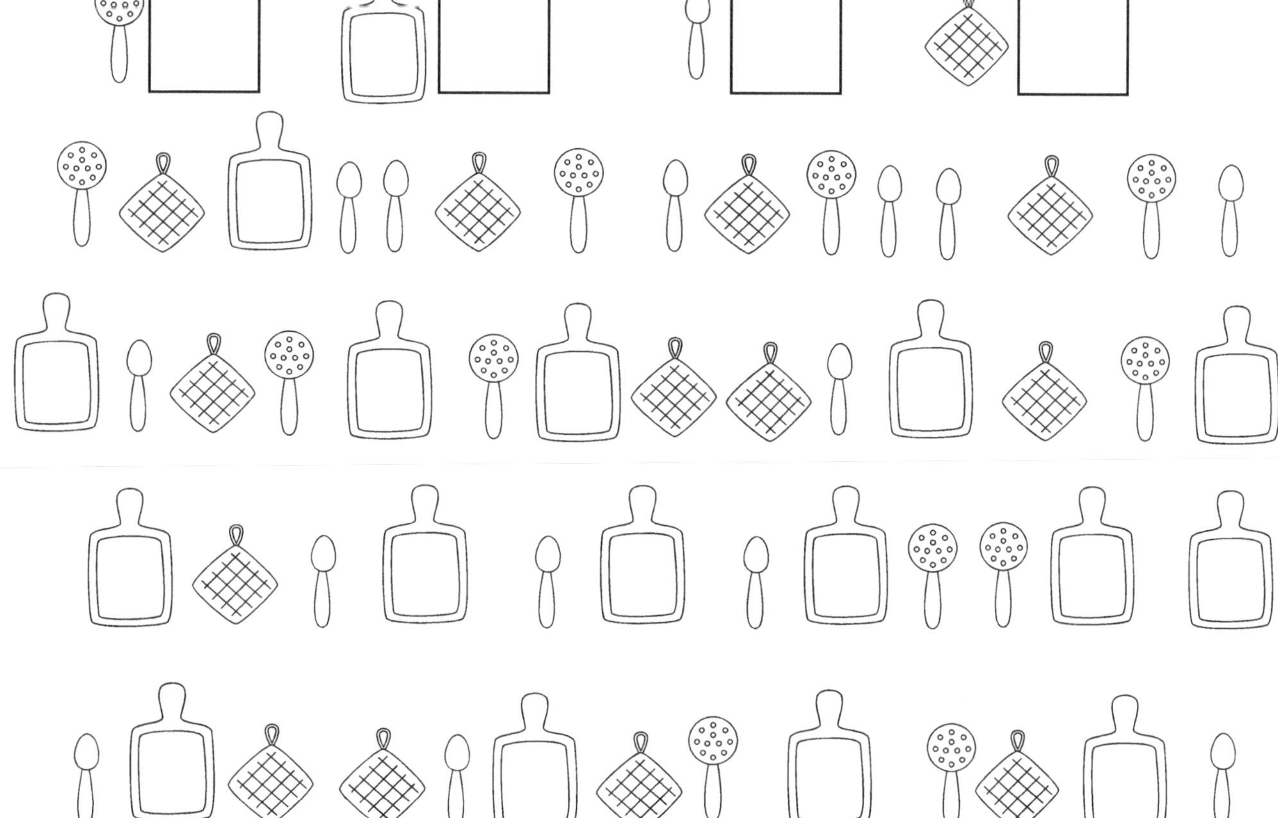

31. Dot to dot.

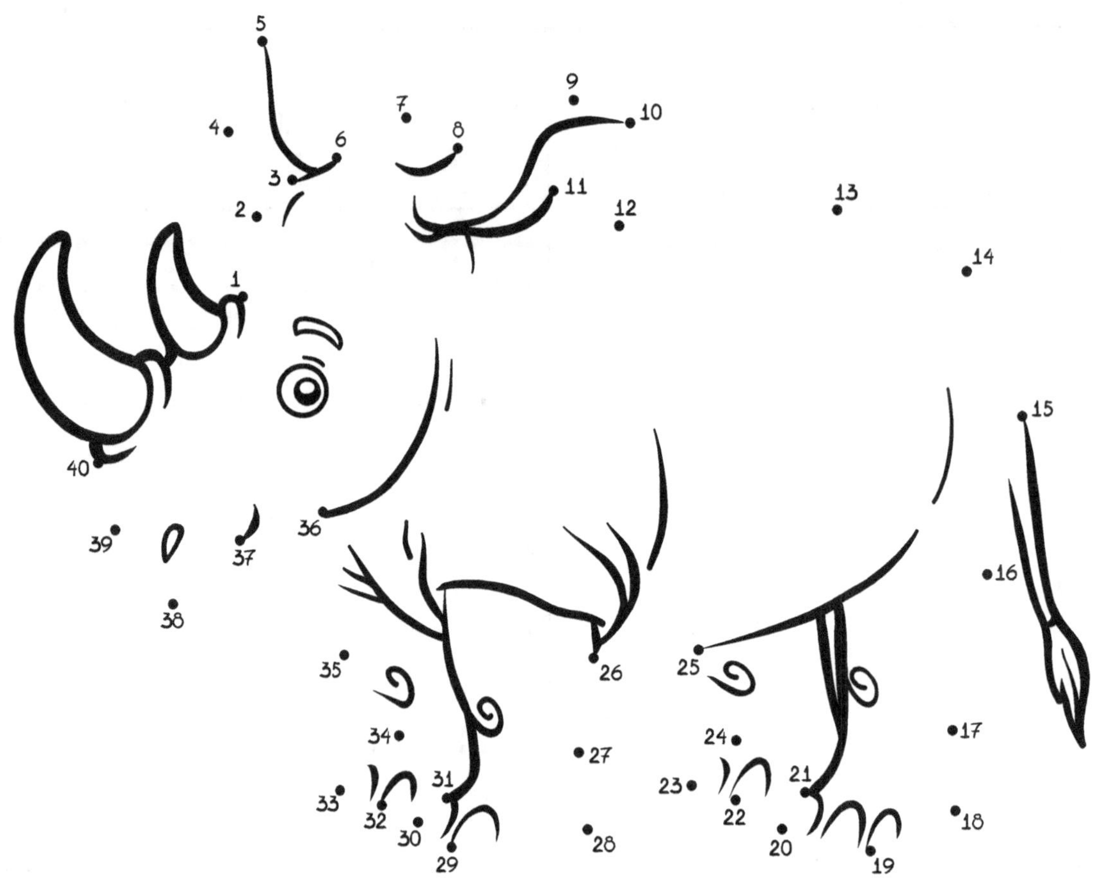

32. Read and remember, cover with your hand and write from memory.

1212 1313 1414	
1234 1334 1434	

33. Write down all the words that you know describing the word - Mushrooms:

....

....

....

....

....

....

34. Matching game.

- 10:04

- 9:55

- 9:45

- 9:05

35. Write down what you see in the picture.

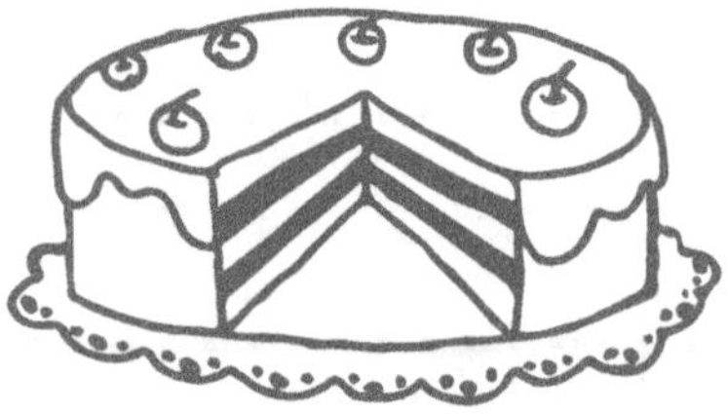

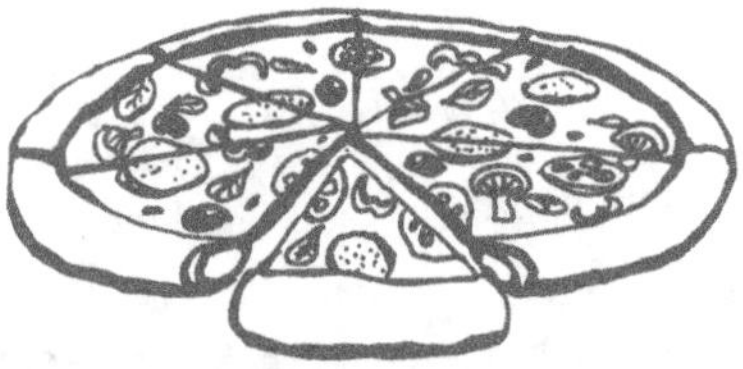

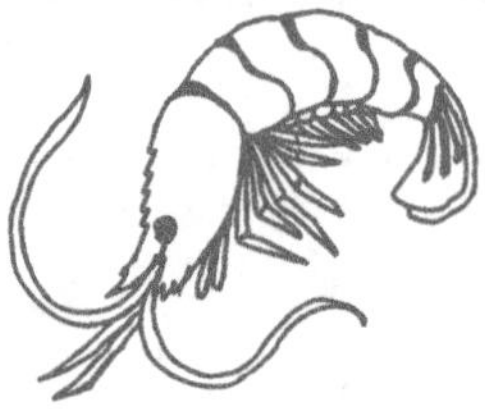

. . . .

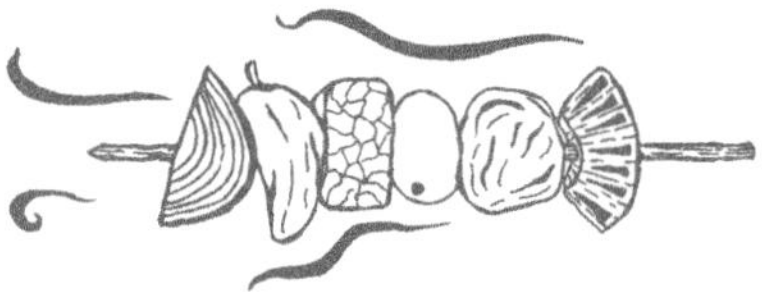

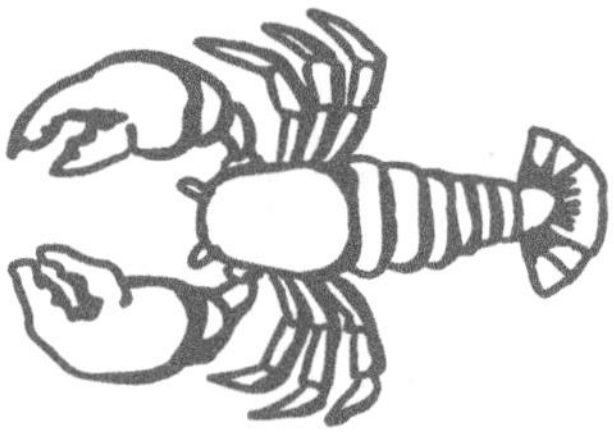

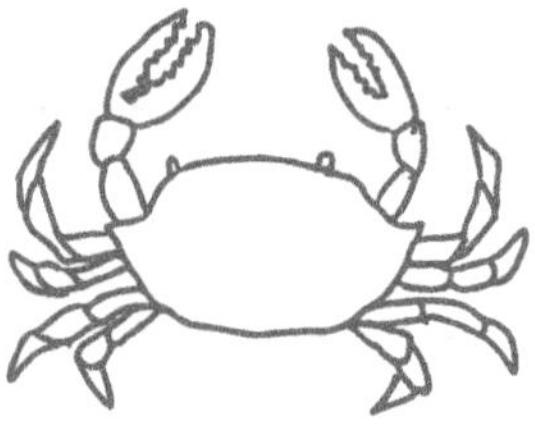

. . . .

36. Copy the picture.

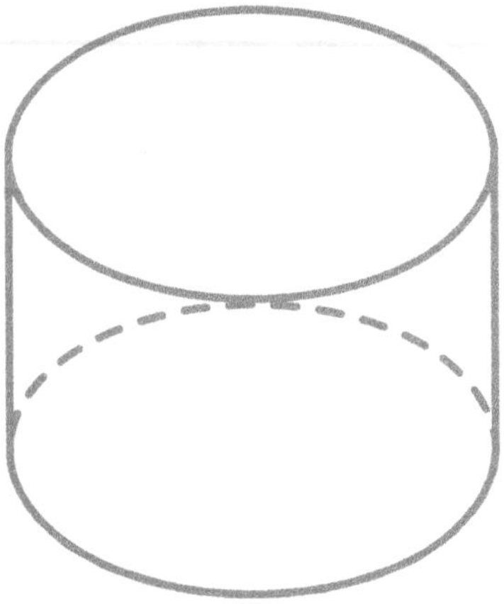

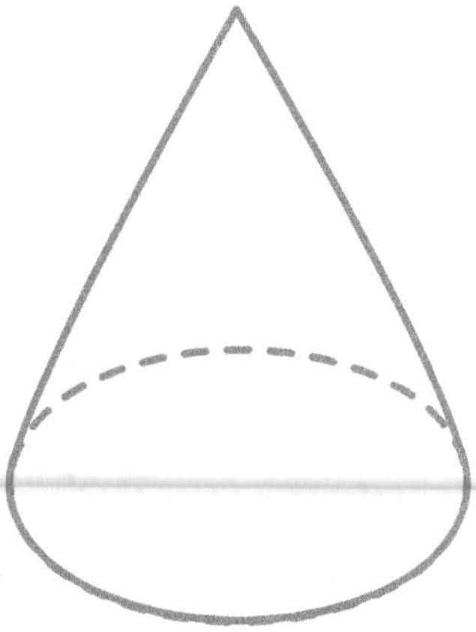

37. Dot to dot.

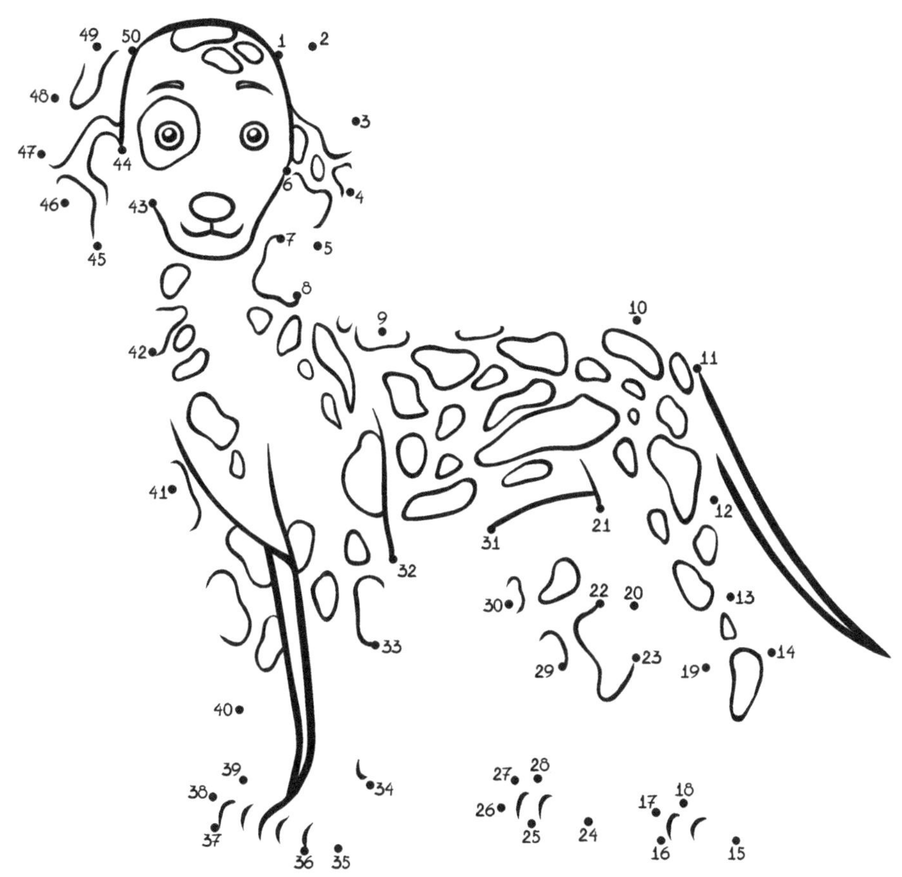

38. Counting game.

4x3=...   6x2=...
5x3=...   3x3=...
8x3=...   7x3=...
7x2=...   9x2=...
3x6=...   4x6=...
12x2=...   11x2=...
4x4=...   5x5=...

39. How many?

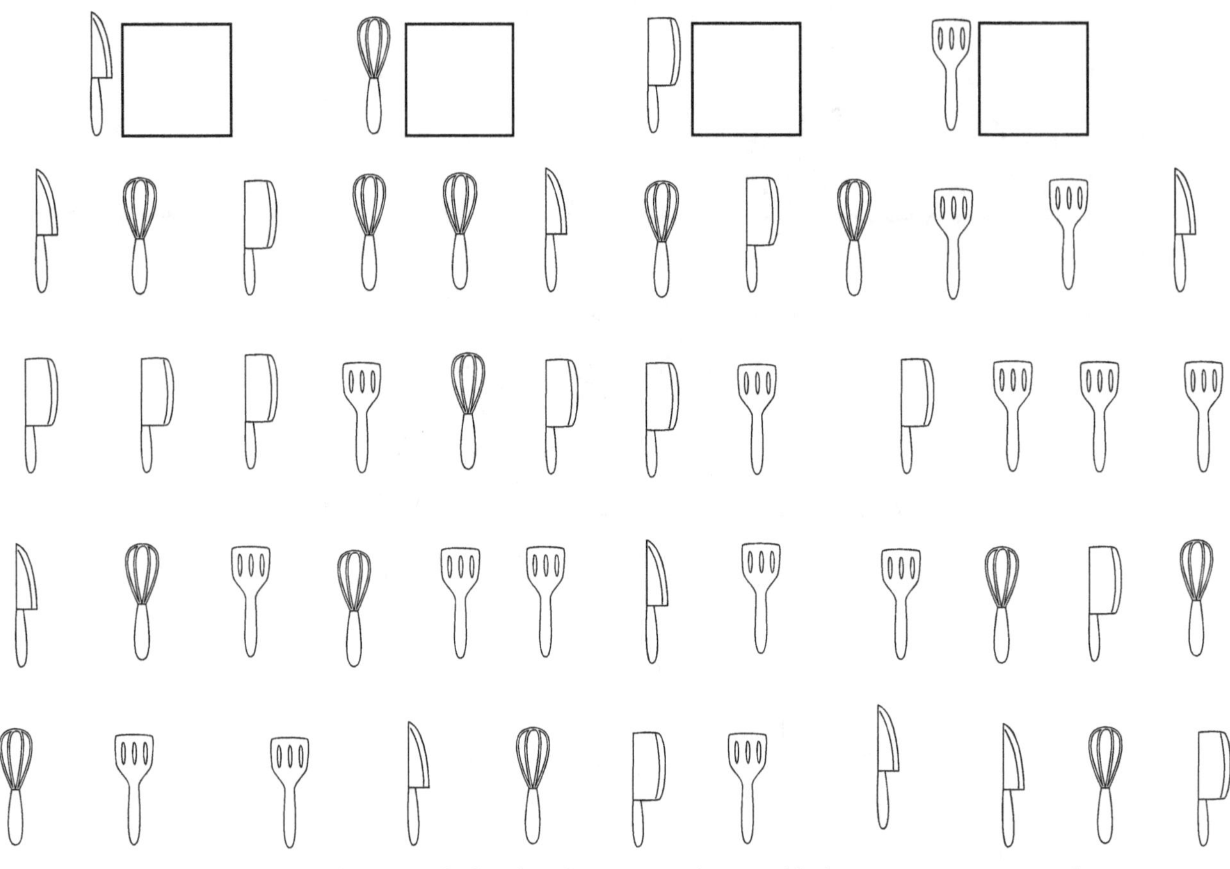

40. Describe your best birthday. Who did you spend them with?

....

....

....

....

....

41. List as many words as possible from the category Jewelry:

....

....

....

....

....

....

42. Write down what you see in the picture.

....

....

43. Number from the smallest to the largest.

1	
2	
3	
4	
5	
6	
7	
8	
9	
10	

89 88 1035 33 204 22 76 4 456 111

44. Find two the same picture.

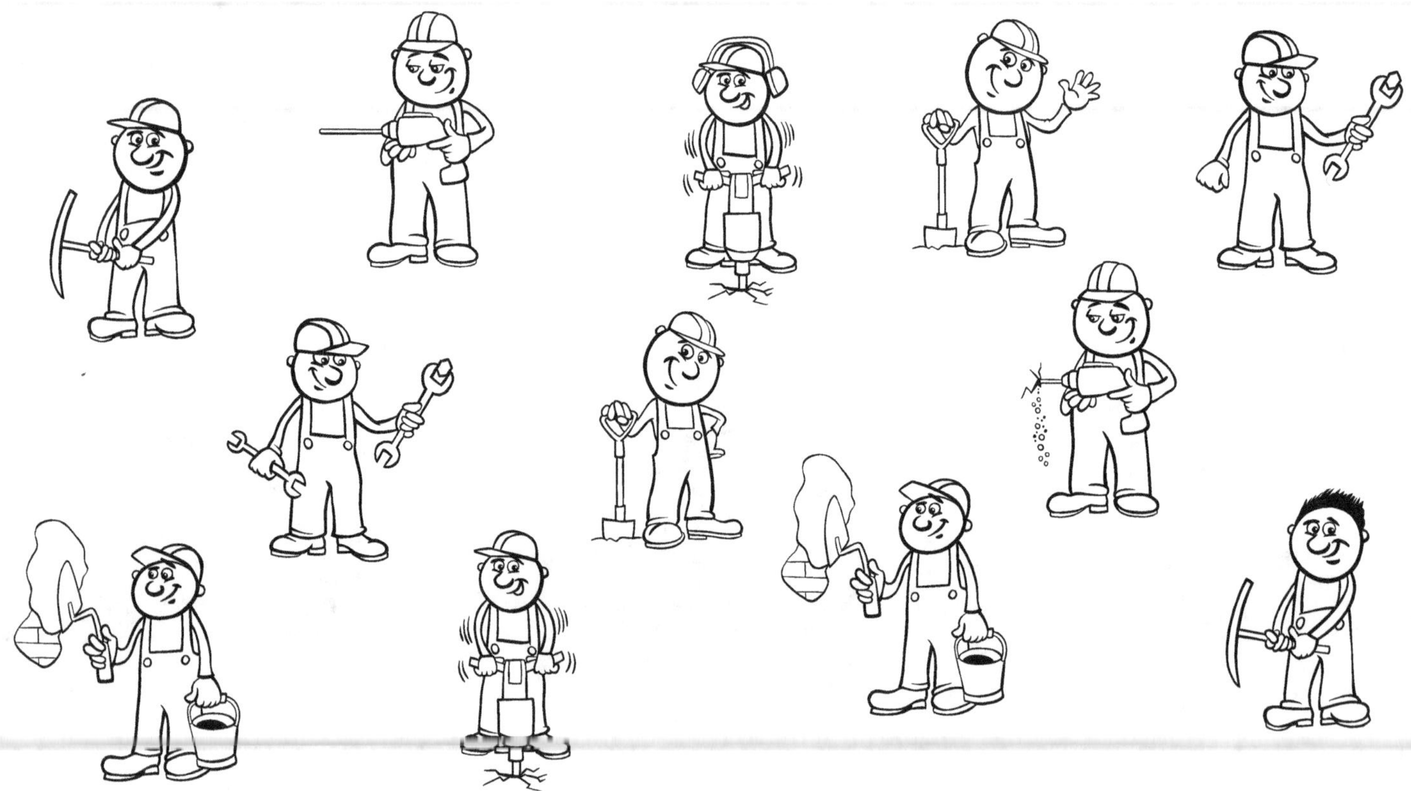

45. Word search puzzle.

H	Z	W	L	P	S	T	O	C	K	I	N	G	Y
E	J	R	Z	M	M	F	J	L	H	F	O	T	V
B	M	E	G	R	E	I	N	D	E	E	R	U	K
X	S	A	D	W	P	Z	C	C	O	P	P	R	S
H	X	T	A	B	P	R	H	M	P	I	C	K	O
J	F	H	T	O	R	T	R	L	H	N	A	E	O
I	J	V	K	C	E	J	I	U	H	E	N	Y	Q
P	R	V	E	H	S	W	S	M	U	I	D	T	S
X	T	M	P	I	E	J	T	B	O	X	L	H	X
S	A	R	U	M	N	K	M	C	K	Y	E	Z	K
K	K	S	G	N	T	A	A	B	E	L	L	C	Q
L	L	K	E	E	S	Q	S	W	Z	N	W	H	H
V	J	X	B	Y	L	H	A	W	K	H	T	N	A
Q	S	C	Z	B	A	U	B	L	E	V	U	Z	R

CHRISTMAS
BAUBLE
PRESENTS
TURKEY
CHIMNEY
REINDEER
STOCKING
BELL
WREATH
CANDLE
PINE
BOX

46. Write down all the words that you know describing the word - Travels:

. . . .

. . . .

. . . .

. . . .

. . . .

47. Find 10 differences.

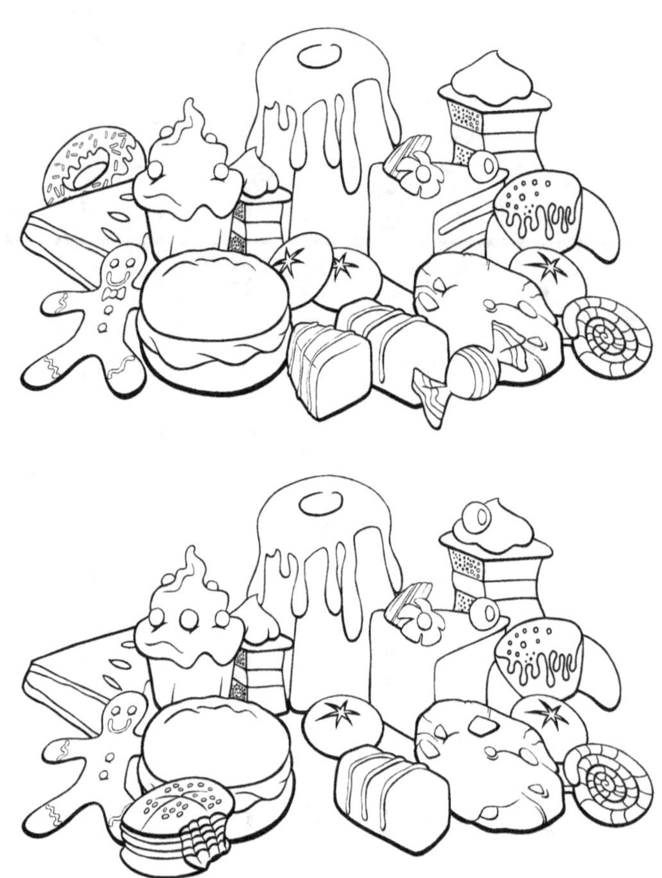

48. Name as many nouns starting with the letter K as you can.

49. List as many words as possible from the category
Colors:

....

....

....

....

....

....

50. Read and remember, cover with your hand and write from
memory.

44 49 94 99	
76 66 67 77	

51. How many?

52. Name as many professions related to the treatment of people as you can.

53. Find and circle the letters sz.

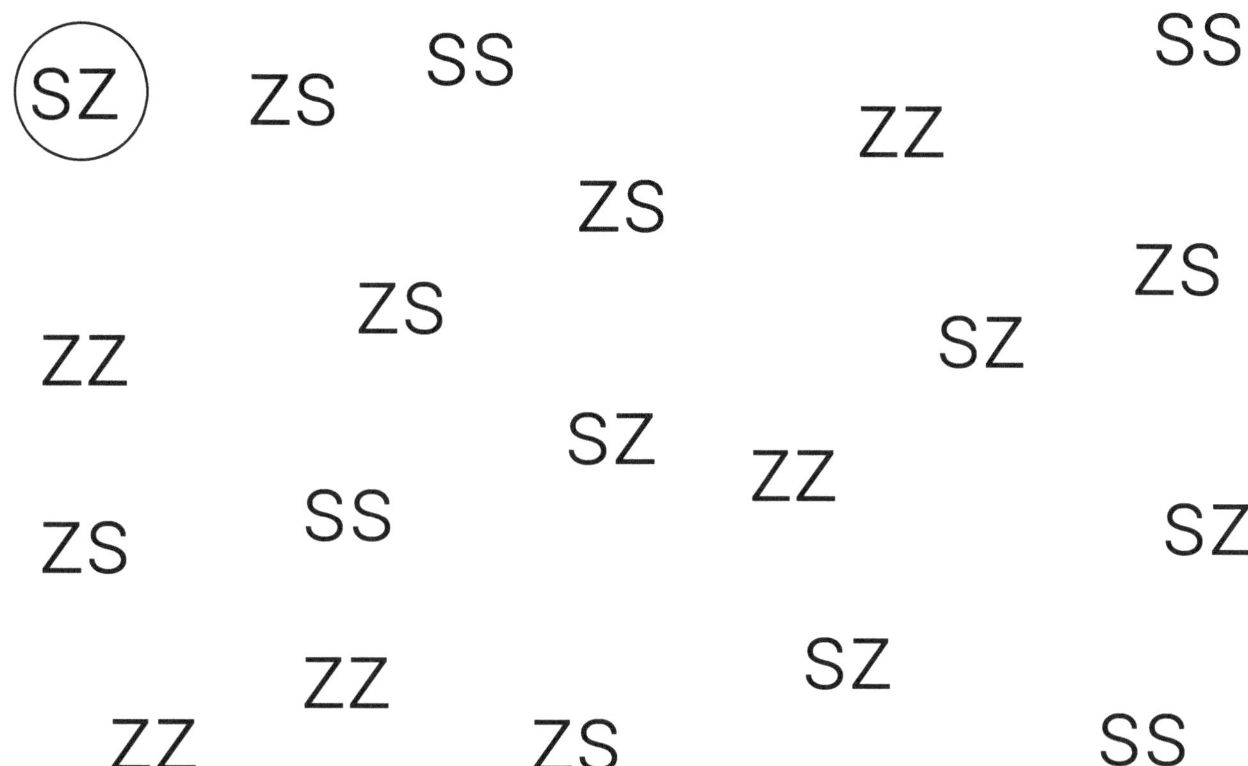

54. Dot to dot.

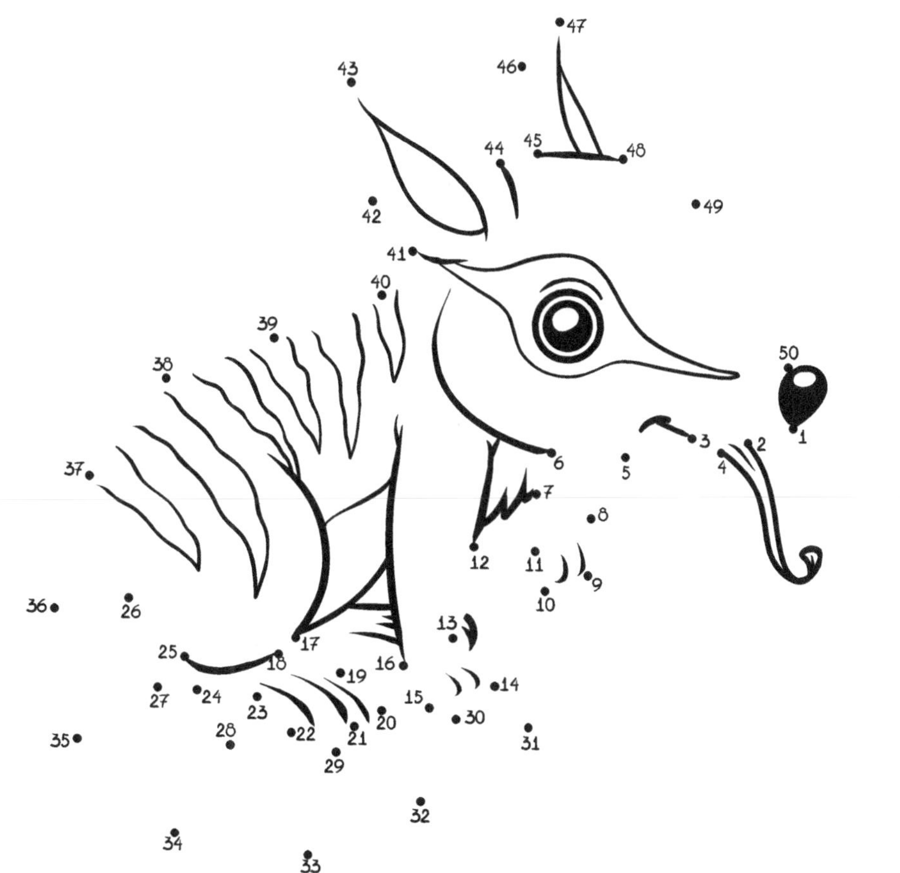

55. Write down what you see in the picture.

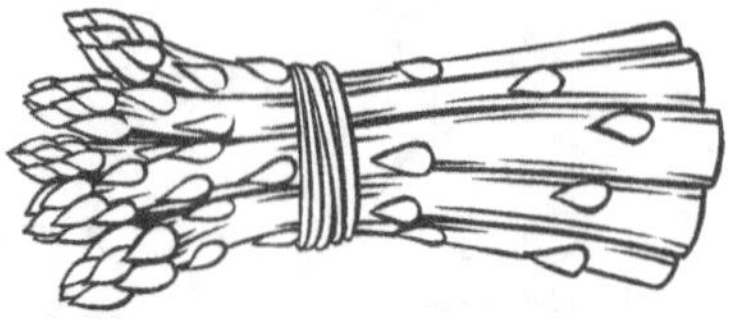

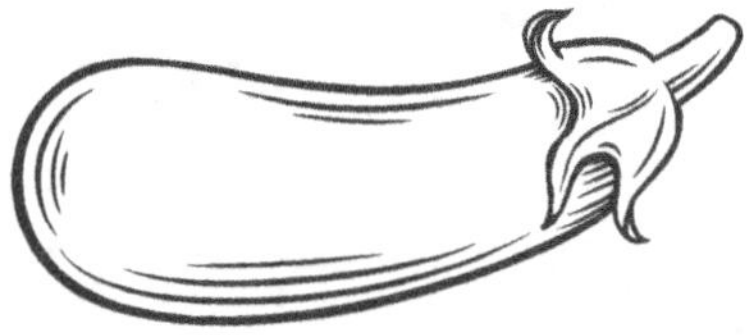

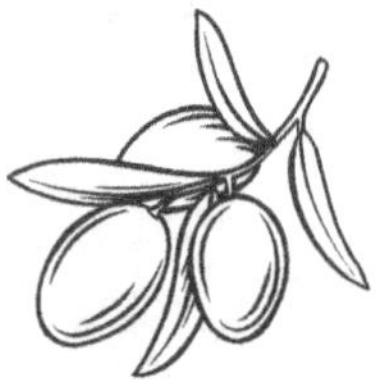

. . . .

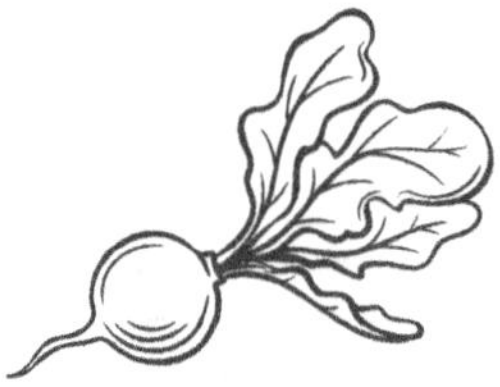

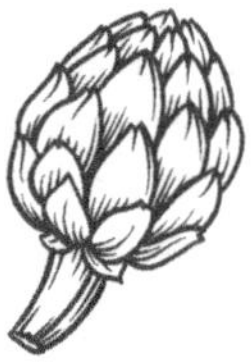

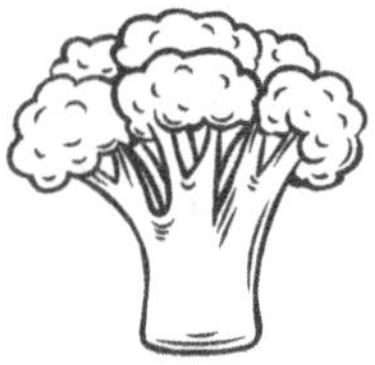

. . . .

56. Name as many nouns starting with the letter R as you can.

. . . .

. . . .

. . . .

. . . .

. . . .

. . . .

57. Counting game.

8:4=...	20:4=...
15:5=...	18:2=...
12:4=...	14:7=...
9:3=	18:3=
12:3=	12:4=
25:5=	28:4=
6:3=	16:2=

58. Write down all the words that you know describing the word - Ring:

....

....

....

....

....

59. Copy the picture.

60. Name as many names starting with letter M as you can.

61. Read and remember, cover with your hand and write from memory.

bread butter cheese egg	
cake chips chocolate ice cream	

62. Find and circle every letter A.

A D E V A F D S A S R I A D F H J K S E F
H P C B H E S F S A A I Z C V N S D G S W
H W R Y U S I A Z C V N H D S D W W A Q
A W R T I O P P L K J S G B N M S Z A E S
S A P S Z F A J S H A I E R U O P C B M A
G W P U S E C A Z S I Z C B N N E W R T I
A W E E R T Y U U J J S D F H J W E W A I
D D F F E R T W E A S S Z C V A R A A F A
S U A S D D S A Q S W W D Y A S D R T Y A A A
E W A Q W W W B H S D G E W W A
K R S A F S Z L H S A S W T U O A W D G

63. Name as many nouns starting with the letter L as you can.

....

....

....

....

....

....

64. What are the synonyms for the words:

Clever	Stupid
....	....
....	....
....	....
....	....
....	....

65. Copy the picture.

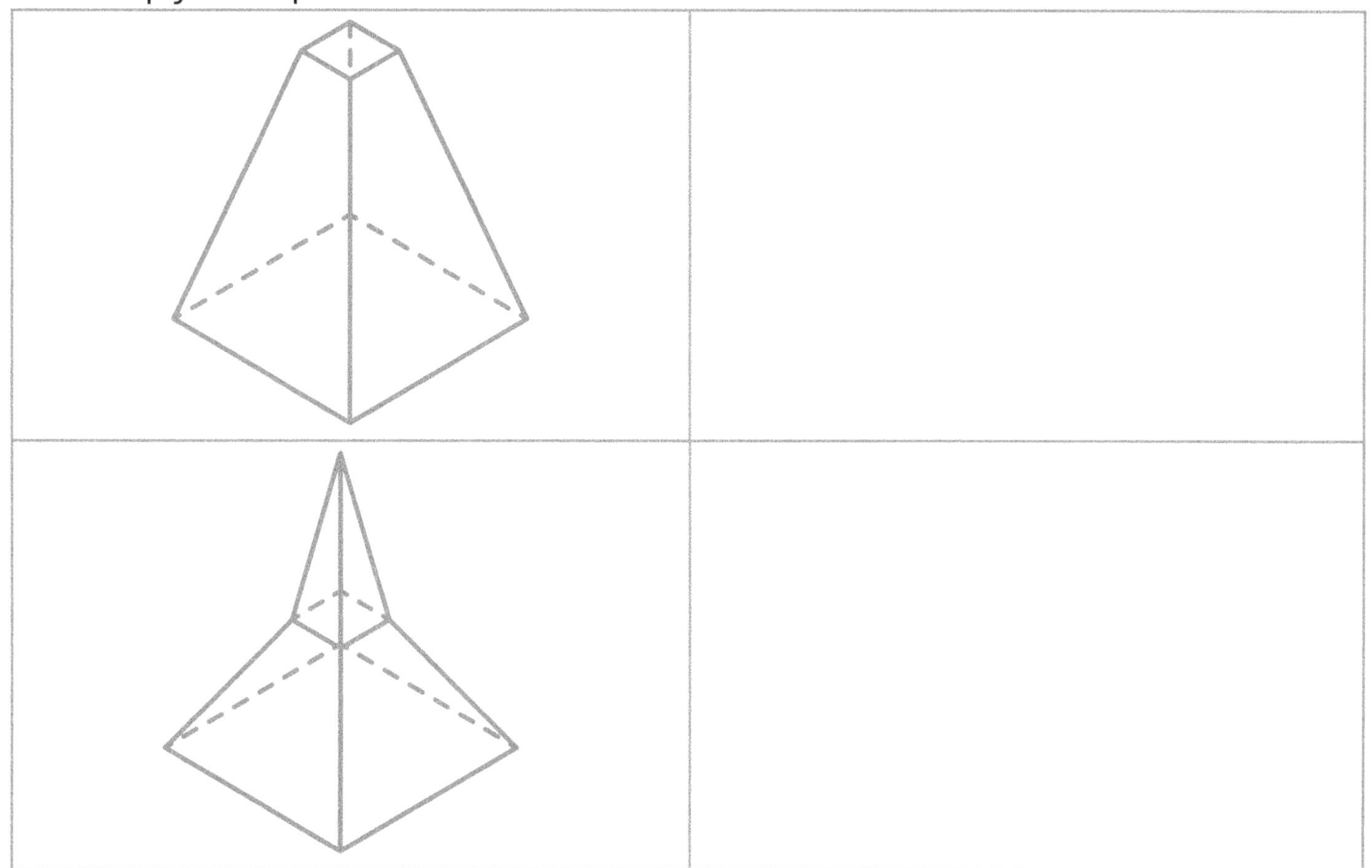

66. Find and circle every letter A.

A D N V A F D S N S R I N D F H J K S E F D S
H P N N H E S F S A A I Z C V N S D G S F Y I
H N N Y U S I A Z C V N H D S D W W A Q T I
A W R T I O P P L K J S G N N M S Z A E J H
S N P S Z F N J S H A I N R U O P C N M A H N
G W P N S E C A Z S I Z C B N N E W R T I A I I I K N E
E R T Y U N J J S D F H J W E W A I U
D D F N E R T W E A S S Z C V A R A A F K J
S U A N D D S A Q S W W D Y N S D R T Y A A A E
W A Q W N W B H S D N E W W A T K R S A F S Z L
N S A N W T U N A W D G I K L O J B

67. List 12 dishes served on Christmas.

....

....

....

....

....

....

68. Write down what you see in the picture.

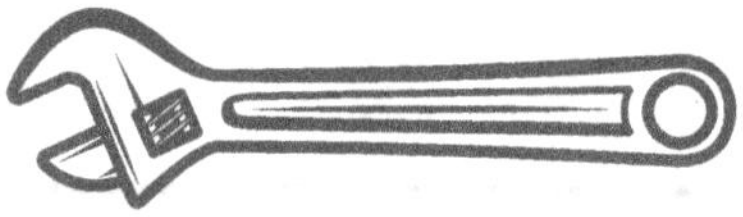

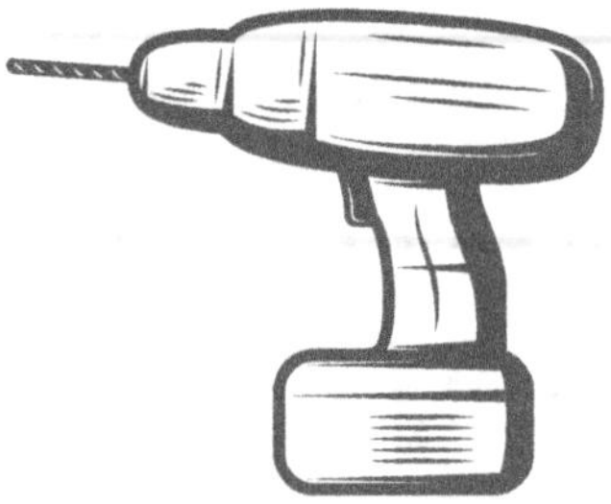

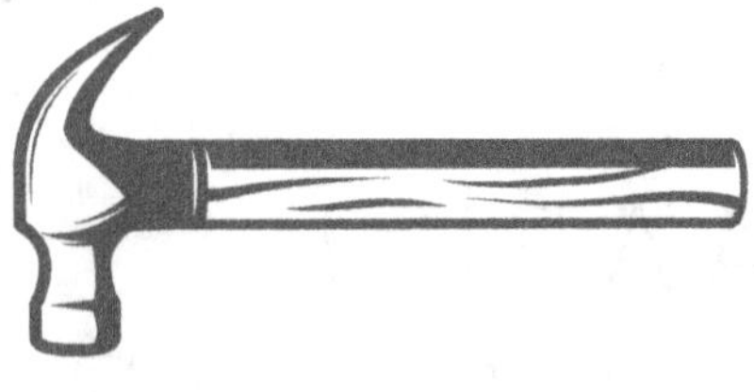

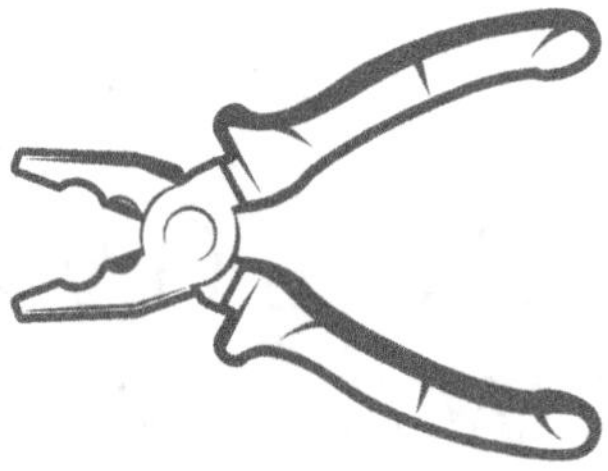

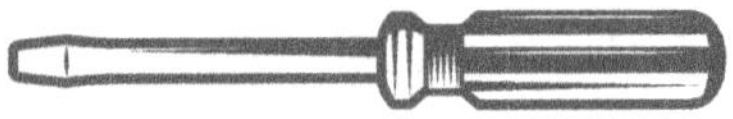

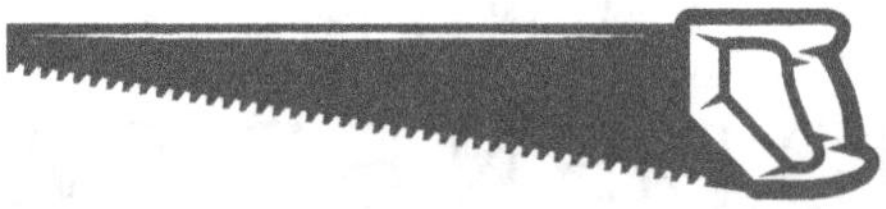

....

....

69. Read and remember, cover with your hand and write from memory.

meat soup vegetable fruit meal	
milk rice salt sugar pepper	

70. Write down what you see in the picture.

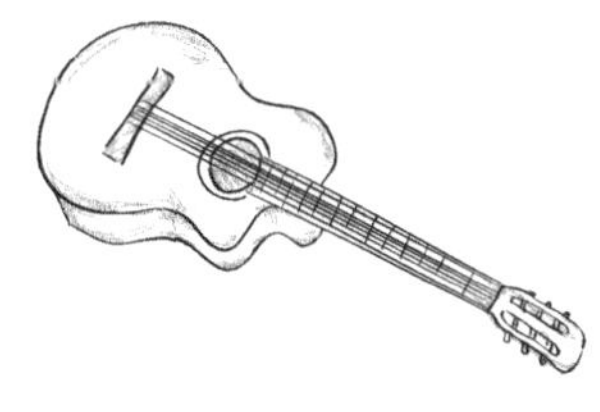

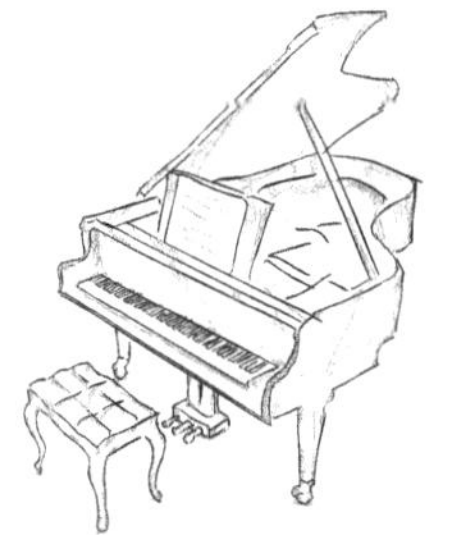

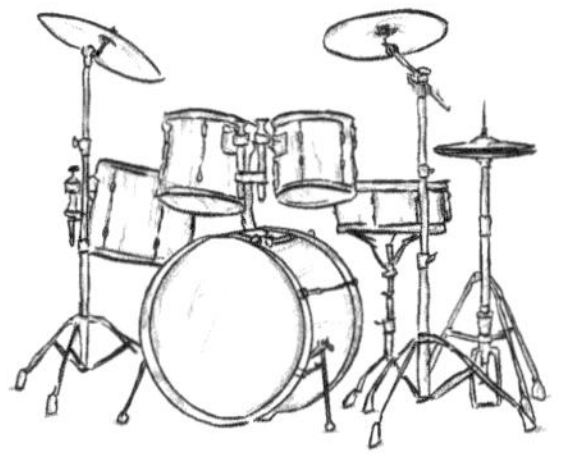

. . . .

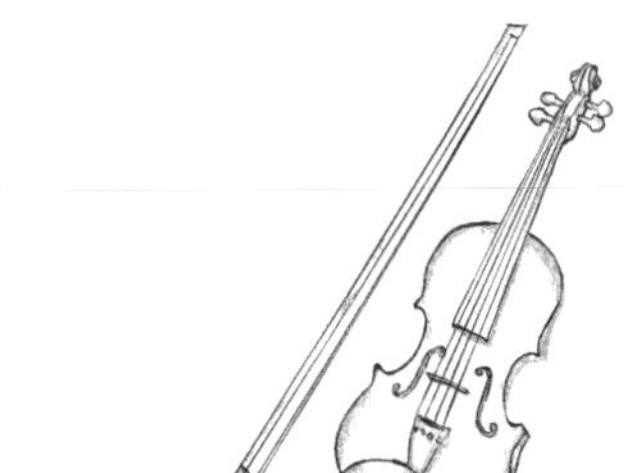

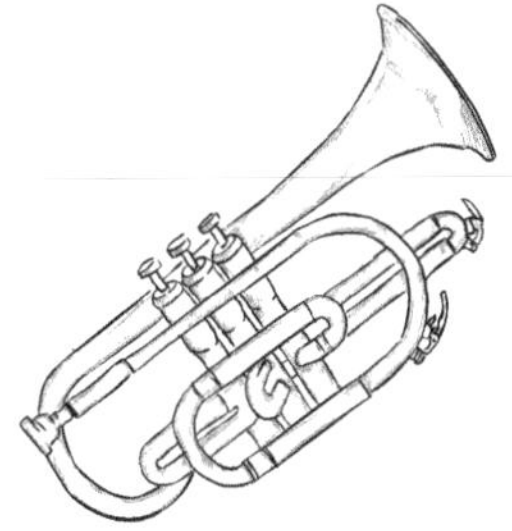

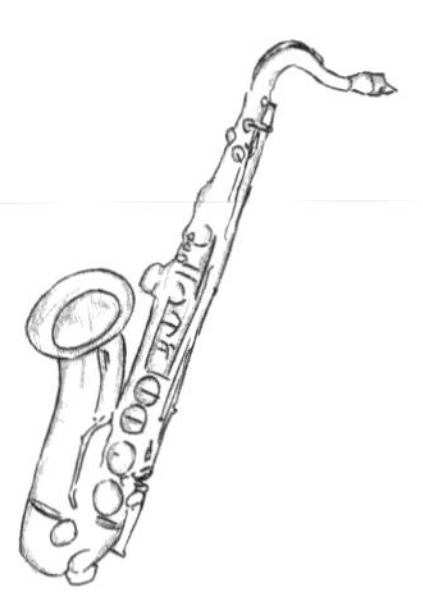

. . . .

71. Word search puzzle.

L	O	T	U	Z	B	B	L	F	G	K	O	O	P
U	E	O	S	I	H	A	T	L	L	T	P	L	C
U	K	P	J	L	O	F	C	J	D	M	N	V	T
M	Y	H	C	T	O	J	A	A	M	Y	C	X	B
C	L	G	C	C	D	B	P	C	X	L	N	N	A
M	G	G	H	S	I	S	F	K	I	H	E	S	N
I	X	A	S	W	E	A	T	E	R	B	M	D	U
X	M	S	X	S	K	I	R	T	W	L	F	R	E
W	T	O	L	N	B	C	R	G	L	O	V	E	S
V	M	C	K	F	L	R	R	R	H	U	Z	S	H
C	N	K	Y	D	A	L	W	R	R	S	M	S	N
Y	N	S	G	R	Z	V	B	V	I	E	C	A	S
S	Z	J	L	L	E	Q	U	G	C	M	E	Z	W
G	F	V	R	N	R	Z	P	A	N	T	S	M	T

JACKET
BLAZER
DRESS
SKIRT
HAT
CAP
GLOVES
SOCKS
SWEATER
BLOUSE
TOP
PANTS
HOODIE

72. Write down all the words that you know describing the word - Towel:

....

....

....

....

....

73. Name the countries of Europe.

....

....

....

....

....

....

74. Copy the picture.

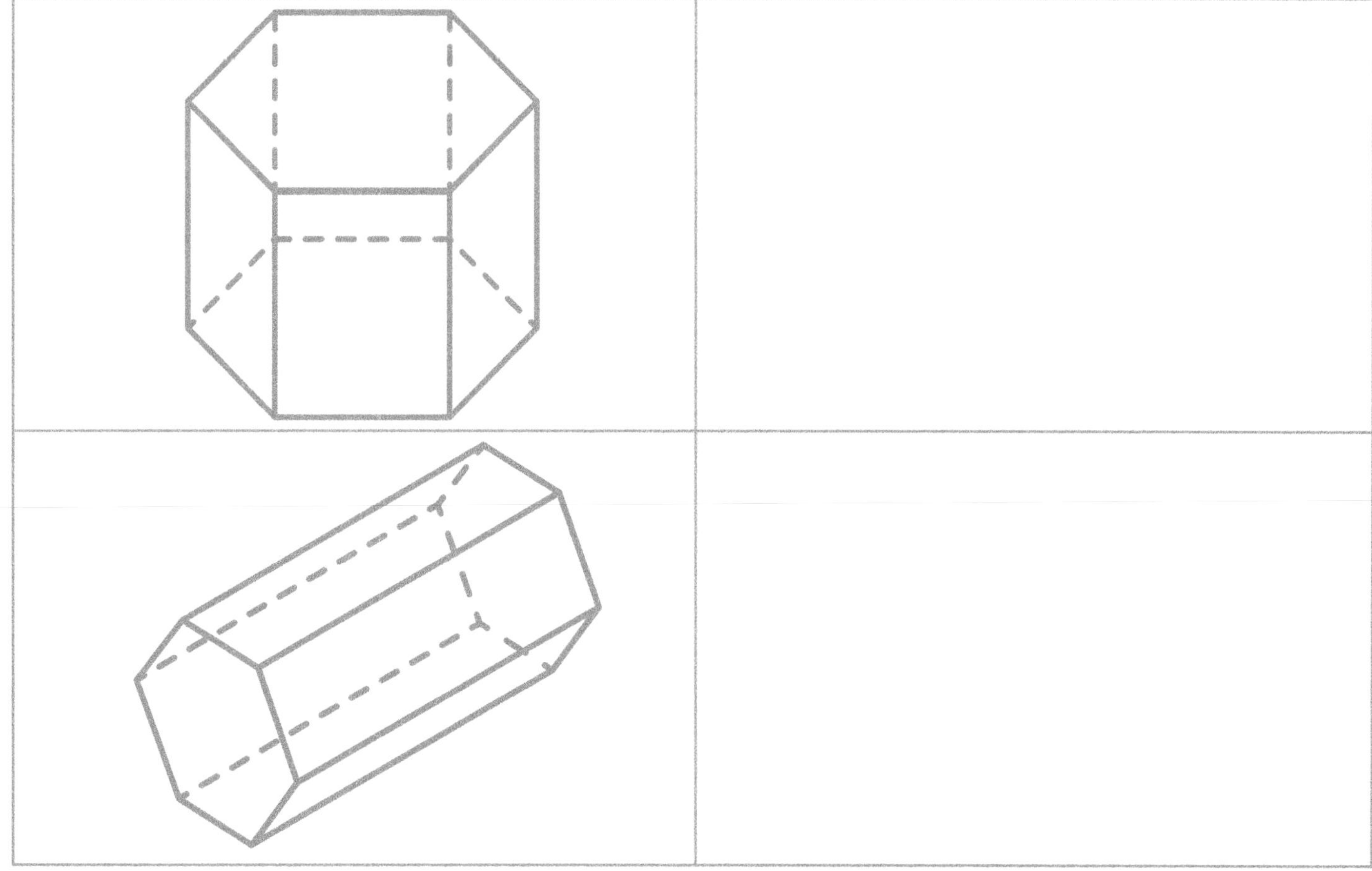

75. Read and remember, cover with your hand and write from memory.

drink glass juice tea tomato juice	
dessert dish fast food breakfast dinner	

76. List as many words as possible from the category Furniture:

....

....

....

....

....

....

77. Name as many nouns starting with the letter C as you can.

....

....

....

....

....

....

78. Write the numbers using words.

11-...

23-...

55-...

12-...

48-...

99-...

135-...

100...

79. Name as many flying vehicles as you can.

....

....

....

....

....

....

80. Read and remember, cover with your hand and write from memory.

house window door fireplace armchair	
bear doll bike blocks puzzle	